# MIGRAINE AND ME

A doctor's experience of understanding and coping with migraine

## Jennifer Barraclough

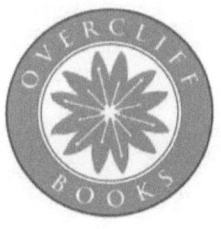

Copyright Jennifer Barraclough 2024

Other books by Jennifer Barraclough

NON-FICTION

*Wellbeing for Writers*
*Beautiful Vibrations: living through medical illness with Bach Flower remedies*
*Persons not Diseases*
*Focus on Healing*
*Enhancing Cancer Care* (edited)
*Cancer and Emotion*
*Across a Sea of Troubles*
*Geoffrey Guy's War* (edited, with David Guy)
*Hughes Outline of Modern Psychiatry* (later editions by David Gill)

NOVELS

*Cardamine: a New Zealand mystery*
*You Yet Shall Die: a psychological mystery about family secrets and a long-ago crime*
*Three Novellas: Carmen's Roses, Blue Moon for Bombers, The Windflower Vibration*
*Overdose*
*Fatal Feverfew*
*Unfaithful unto Death*

## Disclaimer

The information in this book is not intended to replace professional healthcare advice for individual cases. The medical content is accurate to the best of my knowledge but, having been retired from my medical career for many years, I cannot claim to write with the authority of a practicing doctor.

## Acknowledgements

Besides drawing on my own experience, this book includes stories and comments from other people, mainly anonymous. I thank them all for their contributions.

## Contents

Disclaimer .................................................................................. iii
Acknowledgements................................................................... iii
INTRODUCTION...................................................................... vii

1. MY MIGRAINE STORY .................................................... 1
2. WHAT IS MIGRAINE? ................................................... 10
   Definitions and symptomatology.......................................... 11
   Physiology ........................................................................... 14
   Variant types of migraine..................................................... 15
   Differential diagnosis .......................................................... 19
   Comorbidity and complications........................................... 20
   Prognosis.............................................................................. 22
3. VULNERABILITY............................................................ 25
   Genetics ............................................................................... 25
   Childhood trauma ................................................................ 26
   Neurological and Musculo-skeletal disorders...................... 27
   Gut-brain axis dysfunction .................................................. 28
   Female sex........................................................................... 29
4. TRIGGERS........................................................................ 32
   Diet....................................................................................... 32
   Sleep..................................................................................... 40
   Stress.................................................................................... 41
   Environmental factors.......................................................... 46
5. PSYCHOSOCIAL ASPECTS ........................................... 49
   Stigma and misunderstanding .............................................. 50
   Emotional responses to migraine ......................................... 54
   Suicide and self-harm .......................................................... 56
   A migraine personality?....................................................... 58

  Migraine as messenger or metaphor ............................... 60

6.    PRINCIPLES OF PREVENTION ............................... 62
  Lifestyle and self-help ............................................... 62
  Medical consultations .............................................. 64
  Choosing preventive regimes .................................. 66

7. PREVENTION: A-Z of specific approaches ................... 70
  Acupuncture ............................................................. 70
  Analgesics ................................................................. 71
  Anticonvulsants ....................................................... 71
  Antidepressants ...................................................... 72
  B Vitamins ................................................................ 72
  Beta-blockers ........................................................... 72
  Biofeedback ............................................................. 72
  Botulinum toxin (Botox) .......................................... 73
  Butterbur .................................................................. 74
  Cannabis ................................................................... 74
  CGRP-targeting drugs .............................................. 75
  Coenzyme Q10 ........................................................ 75
  Counselling and psychotherapy ............................. 75
  Creative therapies ................................................... 77
  Dietary approaches ................................................. 77
  Energy healing ......................................................... 77
  Exercise techniques ................................................. 78
  Feverfew ................................................................... 78
  Flower essences ...................................................... 81
  Homeopathy ............................................................ 81
  Hypnotherapy and guided imagery (visualisation) ................ 82
  Magnesium .............................................................. 83

  Massage and reflexology ........................................................ 83

  Meditation and mindfulness.................................................. 84

  Melatonin................................................................................ 84

  Migraine glasses.................................................................... 84

  Music and sound................................................................... 84

  Nerve blocks and surgery..................................................... 85

  Neuromodulation devices..................................................... 86

  Psychedelics ......................................................................... 87

  Relaxation training ............................................................... 87

  Spinal manipulation ............................................................. 87

  Spiritual and religious approaches....................................... 88

8.  MANAGING ACUTE ATTACKS ........................................ 92

  Medication............................................................................ 92

  Self-care at home.................................................................. 94

  Hospital care ........................................................................ 96

9.  CREATIVITY AND ACHIEVEMENT.............................. 97

10.  SILVER LININGS ............................................................ 104

  About the Author................................................................ 108

# INTRODUCTION

I am a retired doctor who had frequent migraine attacks between the ages of 15 and 70. *Migraine and Me* is based partly on the personal experience of myself and other contributors, and partly on evidence from published research. It aims to give a broad overview of migraine, including the psychological and social aspects as well as the medical ones. I hope it will be helpful to other migraineurs and their partners, families, work colleagues and friends.

A note on terminology. The word "migraineurs" may seem rather pretentious, and some people dislike it because they feel it defines them by their disease, but I have chosen to use it here because it is more concise than "people with migraine". For the same reason I prefer the old term "common migraine" to the official one "migraine without aura." Where possible I have avoided disempowering words such as "patients", "sufferers", and "victims". I have also avoided using war-like language such as "fighting a battle with migraine" which could ramp up an unhelpful stress response. "Migraine attack" sounds rather militant too, but there is no good alternative.

Migraine is a complex disorder, and a short book like this cannot cover the whole field in any depth. For readers wanting more detail, there are many academic papers free to access online, and websites providing regular updates and review articles, for example:

https://www.migraine.com

https://www.migrainedisorders.org

https://www.migrainetrust.org

https://www.migraineagain.com

## 1. MY MIGRAINE STORY

To set the scene I will describe my own experience of living with migraine. While some aspects of my story are unique to me, others illustrate typical features of the condition.

Growing up in post-war England, I was a reasonably healthy child apart from being a poor sleeper, having bad travel sickness and a tendency to constipation, all symptoms known to be associated with migraine. I started having headaches in my mid-teens. They were attributed to eye strain due to studying for exams and I was prescribed reading glasses, which did not help. Looking back I think the main reason was that when I got home from school in the afternoons I usually ate a big lump of cheddar cheese. Maybe psychological factors contributed too, though these were never discussed. Life had certainly become overly serious and lacking in joy, with mounting academic pressures and an unhappy atmosphere at home. Over the next ten years or so, I experienced occasional headaches accompanied by nausea. If they had happened more often at that stage I would probably have been unable to cope with the demands of going through medical school and the subsequent rigours of junior hospital doctor posts.

From my mid-20s the attacks became more frequent and severe. During those years I was working in a series of jobs that often involved disturbed nights, had a complicated love life, and was drinking a fair amount of alcohol. The attacks settled into a fairly consistent pattern. They usually started around midday with a pain behind my nose, and over the next few hours spread to involve my whole head. As the afternoon progressed the throbbing pain would become increasingly worse and was accompanied by nausea eventually leading to repeated and uncontrollable vomiting, very awkward if it happened away from home. By this stage I was barely capable of functioning, and unable to keep down any food or drink. The symptoms would gradually subside by midnight and if possible I would go to bed with a sedative, waking next morning feeling much improved but very weak. At that time I had little awareness of trigger factors, other than the cigarette smoke to which I was exposed while working at a psychiatric hospital. Later I came to realise that some combination of dietary indiscretion, lack of sleep, travel, or emotional stress often contributed.

My life became overshadowed by dread of the next attack, though it was some comfort to know that it was not likely to strike for at least a week after the last one. It seemed that there needed to be an interval, a sort of refractory period, in between. Rightly or wrongly I put this down to the gradual build-up of toxic substances in my body, probably due to incomplete metabolism of certain foods.

I don't recall taking any time off work because of migraine attacks, though perhaps it would have been sensible to do so. This was partly because I felt a duty to soldier on until my symptoms became unbearable, which seldom happened until the evening. And I felt ashamed and embarrassed about them. I think this was partly due to unconscious beliefs that sickness was a weakness and, in keeping with the macho medical culture of that time, that doctors exist in a different category from patients and do not get ill. Another factor was that I was becoming aware of the stigma surrounding the condition. If I told someone that I was having a migraine attack, their response did not always seem understanding or sympathetic. I sensed that they either dismissed it as trivial, or assumed it was my own fault. It was many years before I first consulted a GP about my headaches, but eventually I became more willing to admit to the problem and to seek help, and then tried many different treatments. A daily dose of propranolol worked to some extent but didn't stop the attacks completely, and nor did topiramate, nor one or two other drugs whose names I have forgotten. The medications that have now been developed specifically for prevention and treatment of migraine were not available at that time. I took various dietary supplements such as vitamins and magnesium, and stopped eating cheese.

By the time I was senior enough to apply for a consultant post, it was clear that because of my frequent migraine attacks I would be unable to cope with a job that involved too much in the way of long hours, emergencies and night work. So it was just as well that I had no ambition to pursue one of the acute specialties. The earlier years of my career path had been somewhat chequered, with experience in general medicine, radiotherapy, general practice, and clinical and academic psychiatry. But all of this proved relevant later on when I obtained funding for a series of research fellowships, carrying out projects about the psychological aspects of cancer. I then found my niche as a consultant in psychological medicine in a general hospital, with special interests in oncology and palliative care. The combination of clinical practice, teaching and research suited me well and my migraines were not too bad for the next few years. Having a happy second marriage as well as a fulfilling job probably helped.

Towards the end of my career as a hospital doctor I became interested in complementary and alternative medicine. While orthodox drugs and surgery achieve excellent results for some conditions, they have their limitations and can cause serious side effects. Working in a hospice with a holistic approach to care made me realise that other therapies, along with improvements in lifestyle, have a valuable part to play especially for cases of chronic or incurable illness. Over the next few years I studied, and experienced for myself, many modalities of natural therapy including energy healing, Bach flower remedies, homeopathy, acupuncture, colour therapy and Ayurveda. I also took a course in life coaching, and explored various religions and philosophies. It is hard to tell whether any of these pursuits helped with my migraines, though of course I might have been worse without them. I certainly found it interesting and rewarding to explore different approaches both to healthcare and to life in general.

In my early 50s I took early retirement from my medical post, not on account of migraine but because my husband wanted to spend the later years of his life back in his native New Zealand. Leaving my job and leaving my home country, at the same time as going through menopause, involved major changes for me and evoked some mixed emotions. But on balance I viewed the move as a positive one. I don't recall being troubled by migraine attacks any more than usual during the transition. We settled happily into our new home and I occupied my time with writing and editing books, seeing Bach flower and coaching clients, animal welfare work, and choral singing. I could afford to visit my friends and family back in England once a year. My way of life was idyllic and almost stress-free, yet the worst part of my "migraine journey" was yet to come.

The symptom pattern changed. I would wake in the morning feeling dreadful all over and have repeated bouts of diarrhoea. Then came repeated bouts of copious vomiting, bringing up undigested food I had eaten over the past 24 hours. And then the headache would start and gradually worsen so that I was confined to bed for the rest of the day. This type of attack was agonising and totally disabling. It was just as well that I was no longer in salaried employment, because I could not possibly have gone to work on such days. I had many similar attacks over the next ten years or so. During this time I kept hand-drawn records on graph paper, using a new sheet for each year, with the horizontal x axis at the bottom showing the months, and the vertical y axis marking the severity of attacks on a 10-point scale. I wrote any comments along the top. Nowadays a selection of "migraine diaries" with varying degrees of detail can be downloaded from the internet, but my rough-and-ready version worked quite well. Looking back at them while writing this book I was reminded how badly migraine impacted my life at that time. For example during 2011, when I was aged 64, I had 24 attacks of which half were bad enough to involve vomiting, was taking magnesium, and had a session of colour therapy.

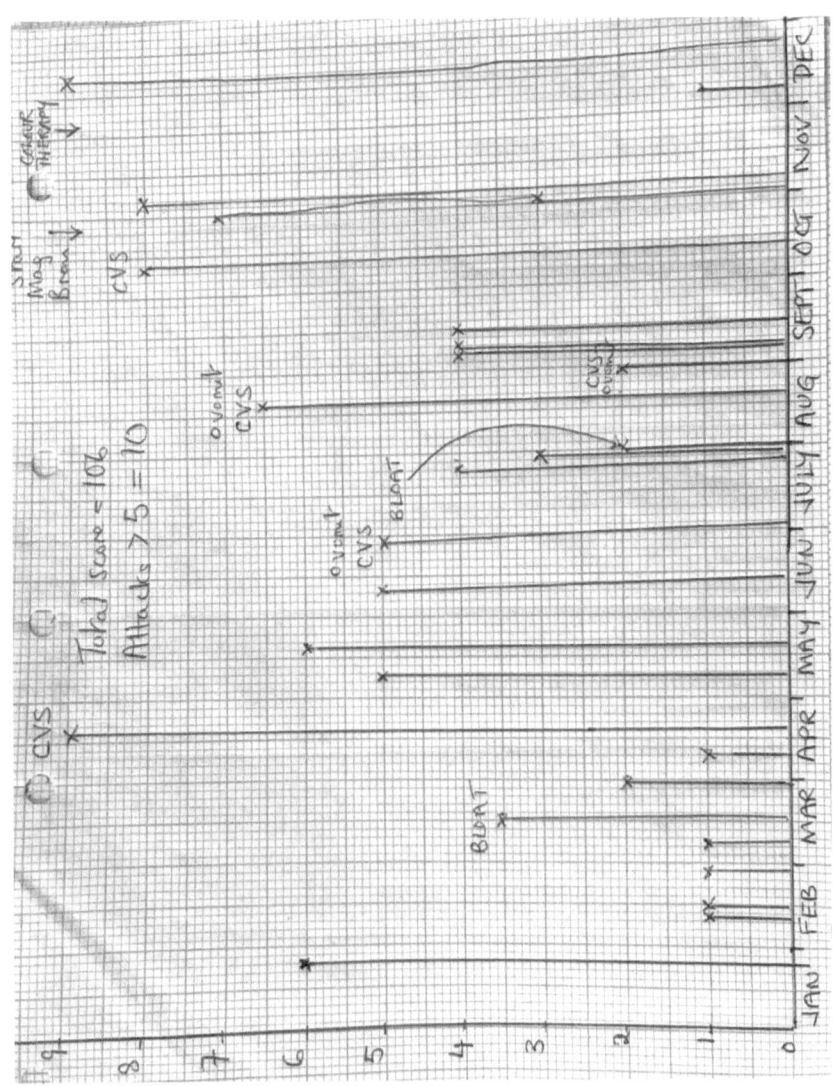

My hand-drawn "Migraine Diary" for the year 2011

My late mother had attacks very similar to mine for most of her adult life. She was reluctant to talk about them but I remember her once giving me some encouragement by saying "Just wait till you're 70". And as she predicted, after I reached my early 70s my attacks began to fade away and became a pale shadow of what they once were. I still get mild headaches occasionally, but they are not bad enough to stop me doing anything, and can sometimes be stopped by a couple of ibuprofen tablets. I cannot account for the improvement in terms of the treatments I have received or to things that I have done for myself. I think it is due to the mysterious ways that metabolism changes over the life cycle, and also shows that the body never loses its capacity to heal itself. Whatever the explanation I am very thankful that, despite being at an age when some physical and mental decline is inevitable, my health feels transformed for the better since I became free of the debilitating migraine attacks. I should not feel too complacent, because I suppose the severe attacks might come back again under certain circumstances, but I doubt whether they will by now.

I know that many other migraineurs have had experiences far worse than my own, being confined to their homes with almost continuous chronic migraines, or having such severe attacks that they need hospital care. I can imagine how dreadful this must be, and although most of these people will have "tried everything", I hope there might be something new in this book that will help. For me, although migraine has blighted my own life quite significantly, its impact has not been entirely negative. It has encouraged me to take better care of my health, and to explore subjects I would not otherwise have considered, and I count myself lucky to have lived long enough to have virtually grown out of it. Rather than fruitlessly searching for the "root cause" of the condition, or for the "magic bullet" to provide a complete cure, I have come to accept the tendency to migraine as part of my genetic makeup, while learning to live with it and looking for ways of moderating its effects.

Jennifer Barraclough, Auckland, 2024

## 2. WHAT IS MIGRAINE?

Migraine is a complex disorder that can present in various guises. It is known to have existed for thousands of years, descriptions of its symptoms having been found in records from the ancient civilisations of Babylon, Egypt, Greece and Rome. Today, migraine is recognised as a serious neurological disorder that currently affects around a billion people worldwide, impairing the ability to work and carry out activities, and damaging personal relationships. Attacks often start during the teenage years, peak in the 30s and sometimes again in the 50s, then gradually tail off and may stop altogether in old age. Approximately 20% of women get migraine, in contrast to about 10% of men. This female preponderance perhaps helps to explain why migraine attacks have sometimes been dismissed by male doctors as the "sick headaches" of women who are too neurotic to handle stress.

The basic causes of migraine are still not fully understood, although as considered in the following chapters there are many factors known to influence vulnerability to the condition, and many others that can trigger off attacks. The present chapter reviews how migraine is defined and diagnosed in medical practice, the symptoms of the different types, what happens in the body during an attack, what other disorders may be associated or confused with migraine, and its long-term prognosis.

Definitions and symptomatology

Orthodox medicine, as opposed to most forms of natural therapy, relies on classifying diseases into diagnostic groups. This enables research into what causes them, and how they can best be prevented or treated, and may also be relevant for healthcare insurance purposes. Diagnostic systems work very well for conditions that can be defined by specific pathological or radiological tests. It is less satisfactory for conditions like migraine, for which there is no specific test. These have to be diagnosed on the basis of clusters of symptoms, and this is not an exact science.

The most prevalent form of the condition, formerly called "Common Migraine" or "Hemicrania Simplex" but now officially known as "Migraine without Aura", is described in the 3$^{rd}$ edition of the International Classification of Headache Disorders (ICHD-3) as follows:

"Recurrent headache disorder manifesting in attacks lasting 4-72 hours. Typical characteristics of the headache are unilateral location, pulsating quality, moderate or severe intensity, aggravation by routine physical activity and association with nausea and/or photophobia and phonophobia."

For an official diagnosis, the following criteria are used:

"At least five attacks fulfilling criteria B-D

    A. Headache attacks lasting 4-72 hr (untreated or unsuccessfully treated)
    B. Headache has at least two of the following four characteristics:
        1. unilateral location
        2. pulsating quality
        3. moderate or severe pain intensity
        4. aggravation by or causing avoidance of routine physical activity (e.g. walking or climbing stairs)
    C. During headache at least one of the following:
        1. nausea and/or vomiting
        2. photophobia and phonophobia
    D. Not better accounted for by another ICHD-3 diagnosis."

In "common migraine", which is the term I prefer to use for my own condition, the headache is often one-sided although mine was not. It may be described as "throbbing like a hammer" or "tight like a vice". Besides nausea and vomiting, and sensitivity to light, sounds and smell, there may be other symptoms including diarrhoea, confusion and "brain fog", dizziness, tingling in the limbs, and pain in one eye "like being pierced with a red-hot needle".

As has often been stated, a migraine attack is "not just a headache", but a ghastly experience involving the entire being and, at worst, making it impossible to function at all. Sometimes the pain, or the dehydration from repeated vomiting, is severe enough to require treatment in the hospital emergency department. As stated in a drug advertisement I remember seeing many years ago "Migraine is hell on earth". And I can relate to this quotation from an anonymous source: "At first you're afraid you're going to die, but then as the attack goes on you're afraid you're not."

Common migraine, by definition, does not involve a distinct aura but there can be more subtle "prodromal" signs that an attack is brewing. These might include food cravings, changes in bowel or bladder function, neck stiffness, frequent yawning, and changes in mood including not only anxiety, irritability or depression, but also feelings of elation and vitality - "feeling dangerously well".

Attacks usually last between 4 and 72 hours and there can be "postdromal" symptoms, such as fatigue and memory problems, in the following few days. Then there is usually a period of complete recovery until the next attack comes. This respite may only be very brief in cases of "chronic migraine", defined as having attacks on at least 15 days per month. In some cases this has developed due to frequent use of medication.

Physiology

What is actually happening inside the body during a migraine attack? Studies using brain scans and blood analyses have discovered various physiological and biochemical changes, some being present even between attacks, but their significance is not clear. One certainty is that the "migraine brain" is highly sensitive and periodically becomes overexcited and inflamed, usually in response to one or more trigger factors. To summarise current knowledge as I understand it, an excess of neurochemicals such as serotonin and noradrenaline is released from the brain at such times. In turn, these substances activate the peripheral nerves, from which other chemicals are released. This results in a cascade of effects throughout the body, with feedback effects on the brain. Calcitonin gene-related peptide (CGRP), produced from the trigeminal nerve and from neuronal tissue elsewhere, is particularly important. The increased blood levels of CGRP found during migraine attacks are thought to cause increased inflammation and dilatation of blood vessels in the brain, and to the transmission of pain signals. Other inflammatory substances including histamine, cytokines and prostaglandins are also involved.

Variant types of migraine

Most of the material in this book relates to common migraine as described above, but other variants are recognised including migraine with aura (classical migraine), chronic migraine, familial hemiplegic migraine, cyclic vomiting syndrome, abdominal migraine, migraine with brainstem aura, vestibular migraine and more. The symptoms of the different types may seem very different from each other, but there are genetic links between them. My husband occasionally gets migraine auras without a headache. He writes:

*I opened The Times one morning and started to read the Leader. Immediately I noticed a shimmering in my central vision. I blinked several times to clear what I thought must be something on the cornea. When that did not work I rubbed my eyelids, but that didn't work either. The shimmering got bigger and a projection appeared on the top and slowly extended to the right as a line of silvery crenelations (these are jagged lines like the structures on top of a castle). After 15 or 20 minutes they disappeared. I* did not have a headache. I was 28 years of age and this was my first episode of classical migraine. I rather enjoyed the spectacle. (A note from me: those of us who know the misery of having "common migraine" may find this an irritating comment). I continued to have occasional attacks, two or three times a year. Sometimes I would see a brown or black scotoma which gradually shrank and disappeared.

My mother had episodes of severe headache with vomiting and photophobia lasting several days when she would have to go to bed. My brother, my only sibling, suffered similarly but not as severely. My father never had a headache.

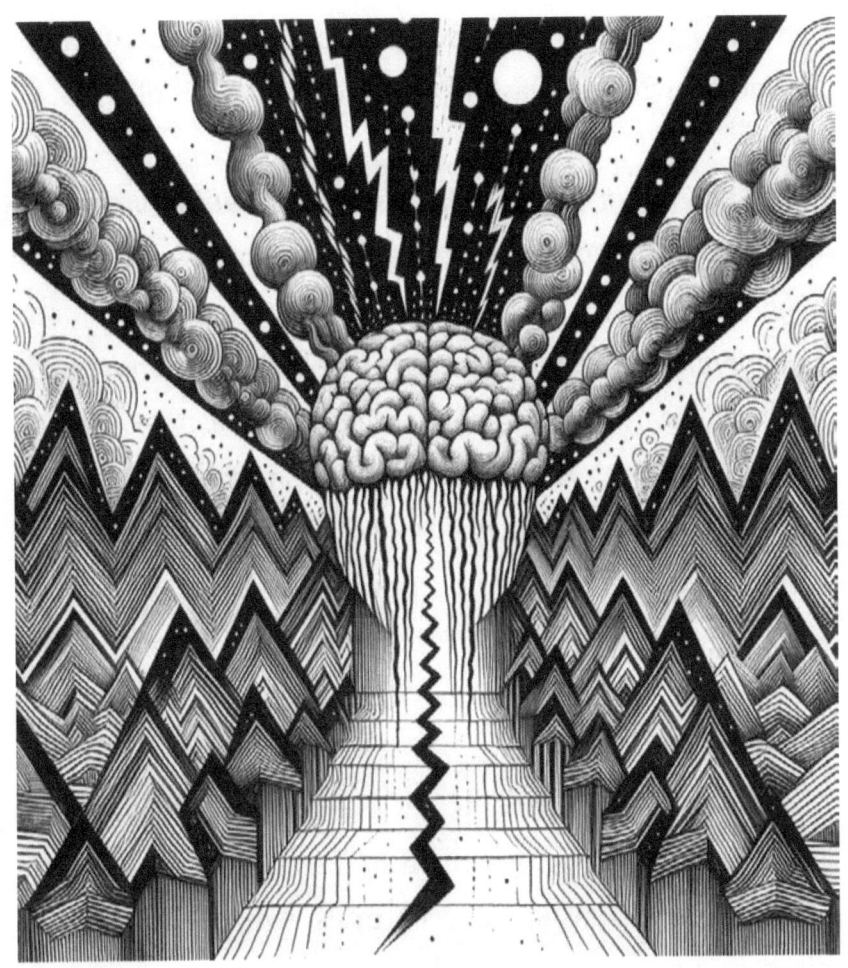
Abstract impression (AI generated) of a migraine aura

In some cases, the aura of classical migraine involves neurological symptoms similar to those caused by a stroke. These can be very alarming even though they usually last less than an hour. Examples are loss of vision, inability to speak, strange sensations or weakness on one side of the body, and confusion. The neurologist Oliver Sacks had his first attack when he was only three or four years old:

*I was playing in the garden when a brilliant, shimmering light appeared to my left—dazzlingly bright, almost as bright as the sun. It expanded, becoming an enormous shimmering semicircle stretching from the ground to the sky, with sharp zigzagging borders and brilliant blue and orange colours. Then, behind the brightness, came a blindness, an emptiness in my field of vision, and soon I could see almost nothing on my left side. I was terrified—what was happening? My sight returned to normal in a few minutes, but those were the longest minutes I had ever experienced.*

The spiritual visions described by certain Christian saints and mystics from earlier centuries would probably be diagnosed by modern neurologists as the auras of classical migraine. Hildegard of Bingen, who lived in the 12th century, wrote of many such experiences. For example:

*I saw a great star, most splendid and beautiful, and with it an exceeding multitude of falling sparks with which the star followed southward ... and suddenly they were all annihilated, being turned into black coals . . and cast into the abyss so that I could see them no more.*

Differential diagnosis

Many other disorders can potentially be confused with migraine. By definition it is a recurrent condition, with at least five attacks required for an official diagnosis. Therefore when someone develops a headache for the first time it is important to consider other causes. These include muscle tension, sinusitis, a systemic viral infection, and hangover. Less common but more serious ones include stroke, meningitis or encephalitis, subdural haematoma and brain tumor.

The challenge of making a diagnosis is illustrated by the following story contributed by a friend of mine.

*A couple of years ago I lost the ability to articulate verbally. It only lasted about a minute and as it was night time I went to bed and slept. The following morning my husband thought it prudent to seek a medical opinion. We were directed to the local hospital where I had all the relevant tests. It was concluded that I had encountered a TIA (transient ischemic attack) and prescribed the relevant meds. Six weeks later when I went for a follow up another doctor said "No you didn't have a TIA, you had migraine without pain" and told me immediately to come off meds. I have never before or since come across this diagnosis and was delighted to not take the blood thinners that caused almost instant bleeding.*

Comorbidity and complications

Several other medical disorders have an association with migraine. There are various possible reasons for this: a genetic linkage, a shared cause such as brain damage, the complications of one condition leading to another, or treatment side effects.

The information in this section may seem alarming, but readers should not be too concerned. Although the conditions listed below occur more often in people with migraine than in those without when large populations are considered, in most individual cases the chance of developing one or more of them is quite low. I have avoided quoting exact figures here because there is so much variation. For example, a migraineur who smokes cigarettes would be significantly more likely to have a stroke than one who is a non-smoker. And the findings of studies carried out in hospital clinics would be different from those based on community surveys.

**Cardiovascular**: hypertension, strokes and heart attacks, particularly for cases of migraine with aura.

**Neurological**: such as such as epilepsy and multiple sclerosis.
**Psychiatric**: depression, bipolar disorder, anxiety, panic attacks, obsessive-compulsive disorder.
**Autoimmune**: such as hypothyroidism.
**Other:** sleep disorders, irritable bowel syndrome, fibromyalgia, travel sickness.

Along with many other migraineurs I have wondered whether the agonizing headaches, often accompanied by difficulties with thought processes and memory, cause permanent damage to the brain. Experts used to say that this was unlikely and certainly, for practical purposes, brain function usually seems to return to normal between attacks. Unfortunately however, the results from several recent research studies indicate some cause for concern. An increase of minor cognitive defects has been found among patients attending migraine clinics, who of course represent the most severe and chronic end of the spectrum. Statistical associations between migraine in mid-life and the later development of dementia have been reported. Migraine with aura carries a slightly raised risk of stroke, and very occasionally a stroke occurs actually during a migraine attack. MRI scans show small lesions in the white matter of the brains of some migraineurs, but the clinical significance of these is unknown.

These findings are obviously worrying, but it is difficult to know how seriously to take them until further research has been done. Migraine is only one of the many factors that can contribute to dementia, and I think it is fair to say that it is not among the most important, and that the risk for any given individual is small. Following the guidelines for a "healthy lifestyle", as discussed in later chapters, can help to prevent both migraine attacks and dementia, and many other diseases as well. And the long-term outlook for most migraineurs is quite positive as discussed below.

Prognosis

The frequency of migraine attacks varies tremendously and is unpredictable. Mine occurred about once a fortnight for most of my adult life, though I had occasional unexplained periods of remission lasting for a few months. I know some people who have had only one attack in their whole life, and others who are disabled by almost continuous headaches. Even when feeling well, migraineurs may have a continual sense of life being overshadowed by what has been described as a monster lurking inside them, waiting to burst out as a full-blown attack at any time.

Just like the frequency of attacks, the long term prognosis is highly variable, but the general trend is towards improvement with the passing years. Some women find that their attacks become less frequent and severe after menopause, or even stop entirely. This did not happen for me, indeed during my 50s and early 60s I had some of the worst migraines of my life, but I did improve after I reached my 70s. In contrast to the many negative aspects of aging, freedom from severe migraines is a very real benefit.

There is more good news. Statistics derived from long-term follow-up studies have found that death rates are not increased for people with migraine compared to those without. There is a slight increase in cardiovascular mortality, but this is offset by a slight decrease in deaths from cancer. Women with migraine have a lower-than-average risk of Type 2 diabetes. And, as discussed above, there is only limited evidence that migraine leads to permanent cognitive impairment.

According to "survival of the fittest" theory of evolution, it might be expected that because migraine involves so much disability it would have become less frequent over successive generations, but this has not happened. Indeed, the prevalence of migraine is thought to be higher nowadays than in the past. The same gene can have different effects at different times, so maybe the genes responsible for vulnerability to migraine confer benefits regarding other aspects of health. Also, migraineurs tend to avoid toxins and dangerous situations, and to take good care of themselves. Therefore, over the centuries, they may have had a good chance of living long enough to reproduce.

## 3. VULNERABILITY

Migraine results from a combination of causes rather than any single one. Many authorities distinguish between the underlying risk factors that make someone vulnerable to the condition, and the trigger factors that can set off an attack. Although there is some degree of overlap between them, I will discuss vulnerabilities in this chapter and triggers in the next one.

### Genetics

Migraine runs in families, and in most if not all cases some genetic predisposition exists. One rare form of the condition, familial hemiplegic migraine, has been found to be due to mutations in one of four dominant genes. In most other cases it is the combination of many different genes, some of which have now been identified, that determines an individual's susceptibility. These genes can be turned "on" or "off" by changes in the body's chemistry as influenced by many factors: diet, exercise, the menstrual cycle, emotional state, and the external environment. So even for people with a strong genetic loading there is a lot that can be done to prevent attacks from actually developing.

The discovery of a genetic basis for migraine validates its status as an organic disease, and should help to dispel any idea that it is just a symptom of psychological weakness. One day there may be treatments to modify the genetic risk, but that is not the case at present. It is perhaps just as well that my husband and I had no children together, given that both of us and both of our mothers had migraine, and so there would have been a strong chance of passing on the condition.

Childhood trauma

There is an established link between "early life stress" and the later development of migraine. Adverse experiences affecting the child directly include physical, sexual or emotional abuse and neglect, bullying, illness, and injury. Others include being brought up in families that are deprived or dysfunctional due to poverty, drug or alcohol abuse, mental illness, violence, parental divorce or death. Abuse and deprivation in childhood can influence the expression of genes, and lead to structural and functional changes in the brain pathways that mediate the stress response involved in migraine. These changes cannot be completely reversed but psychological treatments such as cognitive behavioural therapy (CBT), biofeedback, emotional freedom technique (EFT), eye movement desensitization and reprocessing (EMDR), and talking with a counsellor or trusted person, may minimize their effects. The ideal solution would obviously be preventing the familial and social dysfunction that originally caused the problem, but that is easier said than done.

### Neurological and Musculo-skeletal disorders

Headaches and migraines are among the many possible symptoms that can develop as a result of damage to the brain from trauma or other causes, or in association with brain disorders such as epilepsy. This is a huge subject beyond the scope of this book.

Minor displacement of the vertebrae in the neck (cervical spine misalignment) may cause headaches and migraines by irritating nerves, and by restricting the free flow of cerebrospinal fluid (CSF) to and from the brain. There is some evidence that chiropractic techniques designed to correct such misalignments are helpful.

Muscle tension can contribute to headaches. Many authorities make a distinction between tension headaches and migraines because symptom patterns and responses to treatment are rather different between the two. However mixed forms can occur, and from my own experience I believe that they exist on a spectrum with tension headache at the mild end and migraine at the severe one.

## Gut-brain axis dysfunction

Other organs besides the brain are involved in migraine. The gastro-intestinal (GI) tract, or gut, is linked with migraine in several ways. Nausea and vomiting, and either constipation or diarrhea, often occur during migraine attacks. In between attacks, migraineurs have high rates of GI disorders such as irritable bowel syndrome and celiac disease. There is known to be a two-way connection between the gut and the brain, mediated in part by the vagus nerve.

The gut contains a mass of microorganisms including trillions of bacteria, viruses, yeasts and fungi of various species. This is known as the microbiome, and it secretes a wide range of biochemicals that enter the bloodstream and have an impact on both physical and mental function. The relevance of this is only beginning to be understood but there is some evidence that imbalance of the makeup of the microbiome is relevant to migraine.

Lifestyle measures that improve gut health may help to prevent migraine attacks. The recommended diet includes ample fibre derived from a range of vegetables and fruits. Fermented foods such as yoghurt are also recommended, however as discussed in the next chapter these can trigger migraines for some people. Probiotics may be helpful. Stress management is important because operation of the gut-brain axis is sensitive to changes in psychological state.

Female sex

One reason why migraine is more common in women than men is probably its link to fluctuation in estrogen levels. Attacks often start after the menarche, become more frequent just before and during periods, but become less frequent during pregnancy and after the menopause. However this was not my experience. Other hormones, particularly stress hormones, can be involved for both men and woman as discussed later in the book. The following story indicates how migraine can be linked to cycles in female reproductive life as well as to other factors.

Lucy writes:

*Hi Jennifer, I am really looking forward to your book on migraine headaches. I have had migraines since I was about 20 years of age and I am now 67 years old. The only time that they really disappeared was during both my pregnancies, and then they used to be linked to my menstrual cycle. Following menopause, my migraines worsened and sumatriptan no longer controlled them. A MRI showed a small periventricular white matter infarct,* the neurologist was uncertain as to its relevance to my migraines. Headaches have lessened in frequency and intensity due to prophylactic use of propranolol (a beta blocker) 80mg daily and Nurtec (a CGRP receptor antagonist) 75 mg alternate days. There is definitely a familial link as other females in my family have the same issues with migraines, all without auras. Triggers include too much chocolate or sugary foods, and emotional stress. Stress will only cause them if I do not have control over the situation, I am a terrible procrastinator, but even when the results of those behaviours cause stress it will not induce a migraine. Problems with personal relationships, upsetting things in the news etc will induce migraines, as will anxiety over running out of medication. I carry meds with me everywhere and on the few occasions when I have forgotten the meds, I have got migraines just thinking about not being able to control them. I can definitely think my way into a headache, but conversely I can do relaxation exercises and visual imagery of being in snow or anywhere cold and I can sometimes reduce them. I live in California which is very hot sometimes but it's usually a dry heat. Heat can trigger them, but if I go to London in the summer and it's hot and humid without air conditioning, they will always increase in frequency and intensity. I apologize for the long email, but it was useful to me as I wrote it, it helped me consider all the triggers!

The question of whether certain personality characteristics and psychological conflicts predispose to migraine will be discussed in a later chapter.

## 4. TRIGGERS

For people with an underlying vulnerability to migraine, it usually takes one or more "trigger factors" to set off an attack. This effect is not predictable. Different people have different triggers, and even for the same person they are not always consistent. Migraine is an episodic, or cyclical, disorder and the frequency of attacks is variable, so there may be periods of remission when exposure to triggers does not do any harm, and other periods when attacks happen even though no triggers can be identified. Unlike most vulnerability factors, most triggers are at least to some extent under personal control.

The number of potential triggers is very large. The main ones are described below, with most detail being given about diet and stress because these have been the main ones for me.

Diet

Both the content and the timing of meals can influence the occurrence of migraine attacks. This has certainly been true in my case.
**Food:** Specific foods can be implicated in worsening attacks for different individuals. My own biggest food trigger is cheese. It took me many years to realise this, which now seems strange, but because it was something I

ate almost every day and its effect was not immediate I didn't notice a connection. Also, this was before it was possible to look up symptoms on the internet, and we were not taught much in medical school about the relationship between diet and disease. Cheese, especially the strong aged types, is a trigger for other migraineurs too and this is believed to be because it contains high levels of a biogenic amine called tyramine. This substance is metabolised in the gut by the enzyme monoamine oxidase, but people who were born with a rather low level of this enzyme cannot process tyramine fast enough, so that its breakdown products build up in the body. Exactly how they can trigger migraine attacks is not clear, but one theory involves a chain reaction causing constriction of the blood vessels in the brain followed by a rebound dilatation, so causing a headache. An excess of tyramine can also cause increases in blood pressure and symptoms such as nausea, sweating and anxiety. Other foods containing high concentrations of tyramine include chocolate, processed meats such as bacon and salami, smoked fish, raw onions, fermented or pickled vegetables, broad and fava beans, oranges and other citrus fruits, ripe bananas, pineapples and avocados. None of these affect me in the same way as cheese.

Many other substances have been implicated as migraine food triggers, for example histamine, present in many of the same items that contain tyramine. Some migraineurs report benefit from ketogenic diets, FODMAP diets, or from giving up gluten, dairy, monosodium glutamate (MSG), or sugar.

Gretchen writes:

*Hi Jennifer, as a former migraine sufferer I always like to read personal stories of what worked for different people. Initially I realised I was allergic to MSG when it was put in most foods (prior to full content labelling) and became very careful of what Asian food I consumed. Lactose (dairy generally) was a trigger, tomatoes, anything too vinegary. I learned not to skip meals and not to eat too much because my migraines manifested into severe vomiting, unfortunately something which I have passed on to my daughter. I do not smoke or drink alcohol and only drink a small cup of soy-based coffee a day otherwise I get jittery, tension sets in, my neck muscles ache. Prescription migraine medications did not work for me. I tried many over-the-counter painkillers and only one worked. I still keep a bottle of it in the medicine cupboard. I believe menopause is what changed my body and its reaction to certain triggers. However, I watch what I eat and steer clear of aspartame, limit tannins, eat more whole foods and watch for those sparkly lines in the corner of my vision signalling what I can only call a malaise. That could also be ageing!*

To balance all the warnings about what not to eat, the more positive news is that regular consumption of a diet high in omega-3 has been found to reduce the frequency and severity of migraine attacks. Specific items found to be helpful include oily fish, dark leafy greens, chia seeds, flaxseed, tofu, walnuts and eggs. These belong to the class of anti-inflammatory foods that are good for everyone, not just for migraineurs. This is because chronic inflammation, in which activity of the body's immune system remains persistently high even when it is not required to repair injury or fight infection, is believed to contribute to many forms of disease. An anti-inflammatory diet focuses on fresh foods mainly of plant origin including different colored vegetables, fruits, berries, nuts, seeds, beans, olive oil and whole grains, with animal protein mainly being provided by oily fish, eggs and poultry. In contrast, it limits the intake of processed foods, trans fats, sugars and artificial sweeteners, refined carbohydrates, red meats, fried foods and alcohol. The Mediterranean diet, well known for having health benefits, is similar but more lenient because it includes a wider range of foods as well as wine with meals. It is worth noting that dietary advice from different sources can be conflicting, that public health advice can change over time and is not always consistent with the latest research findings, and what suits one person may not suit another. Long-term follow-up studies suggest that a balanced diet including all food groups is best for health, and that excluding certain items unless there are sound medical reasons to do so can have adverse consequences.

**Alcohol:** Alcoholic drinks are often blamed for precipitating migraine attacks. This may not be due just to the alcohol itself but also to the various other chemicals, including tyramine, they contain. Some current authorities advise that alcohol is a poison that nobody should be drinking anyway, but my understanding from several well-conducted studies is that a low-to-moderate intake does no harm and may protect against cardiovascular disease. I am glad to say that having a glass of white or rose with meals on most evenings does not trigger migraine attacks for me, in fact it is probably helpful because of its relaxing effect. But although red wine is said to be better for protecting cardiovascular health, it does not suit me so well and is notorious for provoking headaches even in people without migraine, probably because of its quercetin content. I seldom drink more than one glass of anything nowadays, having found in the past that just a slight excess can be followed by a whole day of feeling very ill with a ghastly mixture of migraine and hangover symptoms.

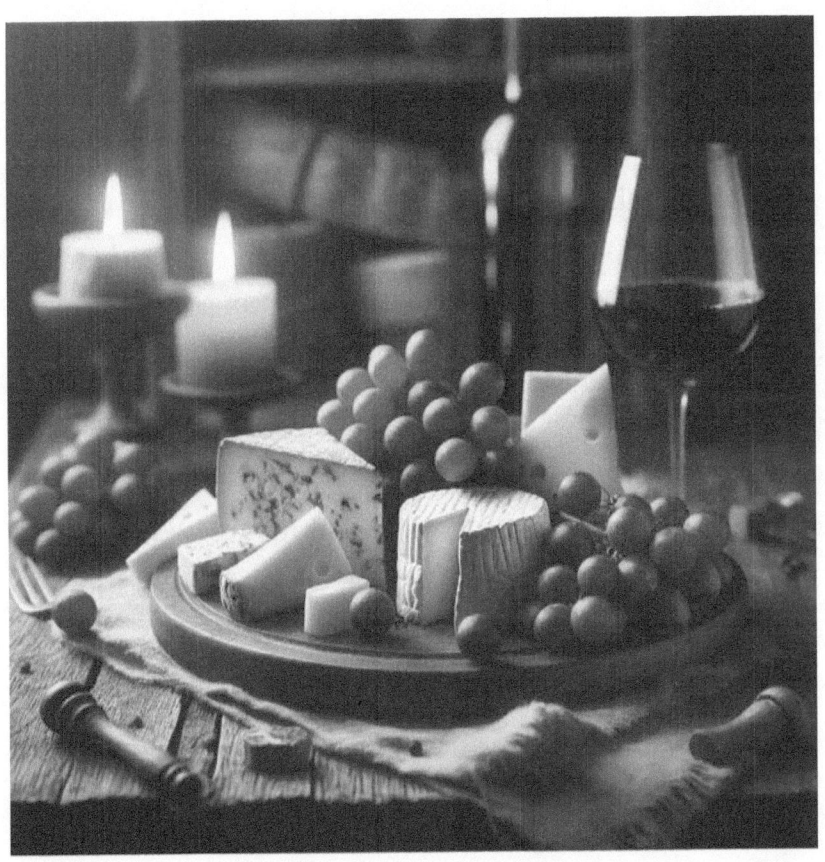
Cheese and wine parties were a bad idea for me.

**Coffee:** A minority of migraineurs identify coffee, and other caffeinated drinks, as a trigger especially if they drink too much of them. Paradoxically, caffeine can also be used to treat migraines. It is present in some over-the-counter medicines, and drinking black coffee during attacks can be helpful for people who do not usually drink it at all. Sudden withdrawal of caffeine can lead to a migraine attack, so it is best to keep a fairly constant daily intake. I am fine with one double shot flat white or long black mid-morning. A few years ago I spent a week at a health resort where coffee was forbidden. I had cut down on it the week before but still had a nasty headache for the first three days, though this did not develop into a full-blown migraine. By the way coffee has a number of proven health benefits, so except for people who cannot tolerate caffeine I see no point in giving it up.

**Meal patterns:** Migraine attacks can be triggered by going too long without food or water, but also by eating too much at one time, so it is important to follow a regular meal schedule and to avoid dehydration. Intermittent fasting is currently in vogue, mainly as a means of weight loss, but may not be a suitable practice for migraineurs because the consequent hypoglycemia often causes headaches. Some of the Christian saints who described seeing visions, whether divine or demonic, may actually have been experiencing migraine auras after fasting for religious reasons.

Food triggers are not easy to pinpoint because there can be a delay of hours or even days before their effects develop. More objective methods of identifying food triggers include elimination diets, and blood tests for IgG antibodies against certain items, but these are not widely used. If someone gets a migraine soon after eating a certain food, they may develop a fear of that item and avoid it in future even though the association was in fact coincidental and played no role in causing the attack. Psychological factors can be important. As regards the role of cheese as a trigger for my own attacks, although there is a biological basis for this due to the tyramine content, I am sure the effect has been magnified by my beliefs and expectations. The very first time I saw a doctor about my migraines he told me in no uncertain terms that they were caused by eating cheese, and this made a deep impression. Even now that my migraines are only mild and I do allow myself to eat some cheese, I tend to worry afterwards that it will bring on an attack, and it may well be that my anxiety and negative expectations will contribute to a headache. This is equivalent to the "nocebo effect" found in drug trials, with patients being more likely to develop adverse side effects if they were warned about them beforehand.

Avoiding all possible food triggers, alcohol and caffeine requires strong willpower, is awkward in social situations, and takes away much of the pleasure in life for those who enjoy food and drink. Some of the "migraine diets" to be found on the internet appear impossibly restrictive and could cause nutritional deficiencies in the long term. Dietary migraine triggers are not the same as allergies in which eating even a trace of a certain food, peanuts for example, is quickly followed by a severe reaction or even death. Many migraineurs can get away with eating their trigger foods in small amounts occasionally, provided they are not exposed to other risk factors at the same time. Now that my own migraines are so much better, I am more relaxed about eating a wider range of foods and feel healthier for it. Looking back, I probably continued to restrict my diet longer than was necessary.

Sleep

Both lack of sleep and, less often, too much sleep can lead to an attack. Like many migraineurs, I have always been prone to insomnia. This was worse when I was working in medicine, being on call for emergencies at night, and – being by nature an owl rather than a lark – having to get up early for clinics and ward rounds. Some people are able to manage their migraine attacks by taking a nap, and feel better when they wake up. This was not an option for me because I can never take naps anyway, and find sleep impossible in the presence of headache and nausea. I now try to keep to consistent times both for going to bed and for getting up. In recent years my sleep pattern has improved, along with the lessening of my migraines.

Stress

Stress is known to contribute to many medical disorders presumably because of the impact of "stress hormones" such as adrenaline and cortisol, generated through the sympathetic nervous system, upon the body and brain. Many migraineurs cite stress as their top trigger factor. Others vehemently deny that their attacks have any connection with stress at all, perhaps wanting to dispel the notion that migraine is "all in the mind" rather than a real disease. Some of my own attacks have clearly been induced by stress, whereas others have apparently come out of the blue. It is too easy for other people to say of migraine or any other medical condition "It's due to stress" or worse "It's *just* due to stress", when this may not be the case at all and is certainly not the whole story.

Feelings of stress are usually blamed on outside circumstances, the negative events and ongoing difficulties that are an inevitable part of life. But it is individual responses that determine how stressful these experiences are perceived to be. Responses depend on mental attitudes, past experiences and physical constitution. There is evidence that the sympathetic nervous system tends to be overactive in migraineurs, causing them to live in a state of chronic low-grade physiological stress, perhaps without knowing it. This would explain why therapies that promote relaxation, such as biofeedback, are effective for migraine prevention. Even when there is no external cause for stress it can be generated internally, for example by setting oneself unrealistically tight deadlines or high standards, or through negative attitudes and emotions such as anxiety, depression, hopelessness and guilt, whether these have arisen in response to migraine or for other reasons. This topic will be considered further in the chapter about psychosocial aspects.

The present section is focused on external stress, and a very common source of this in today's world is an accumulation of the apparently trivial hassles and demands of everyday life – juggling jobs, household and family responsibilities, long working hours, financial strain, traffic jams, a deluge of emails and news and social media posts. Pressure can intensify at times that are supposed to be enjoyable, such as holidays or Christmas, when organising the preparations is combined with changes to routine and possibly with lack of sleep, unfamiliar foods or missed meals, and excessive exertion. People who are continually trying to help and please others, often from a sense of obligation rather than genuine goodwill, are especially prone to stress of this kind especially if they are neglecting their own needs and resenting it.

Feeling trapped in an unsatisfying, or frankly toxic, work situation or relationship is another source of stress. One woman described having gradually come to realise that her physical and mental health was being damaged by the "negative energy" generated by certain family members, and that her relationship with these people was triggering her migraines. She decided to cut off contact with them. Immediately after doing so she developed a very severe attack, but has had no more since.

Migraine itself is a potent source of stress, and vicious circles can develop, as in the case of someone who is worn out after a busy period at work, gets a severe migraine and has to take a few days off. There is nobody else to cover for them, so on returning they find a backlog of tasks has built up so that the workload intensifies, and leads to another attack. After this scenario has been repeated a few times they either lose their job because of being unreliable, or feel compelled to resign, and then experience the stress of unemployment and financial hardship.

The relationship between stress and migraine is not straightforward, and may seem paradoxical. Although migraines sometimes do begin following a highly stressful event, the opposite can also be true; the major crises and privations in life do not necessarily trigger attacks, and might even protect against them. A woman once told me that her severe and frequent attacks had stopped for one year following the sudden death of her child. I experienced something similar a few years ago when my husband was critically ill at the same time that my mother was dying. Although I became unwell myself with both mental and physical symptoms during this period, I did not get any migraines. Others have commented on this phenomenon, for example from Joan Didion's 1968 essay *In Bed*:

*Tell me that my house is burned down, my husband has left me, that there is gunfighting in the streets and panic in the banks, and I will not respond by getting a headache. It comes instead when I am fighting not an open but a guerrilla war with my own life, during weeks of small household confusions, lost laundry, unhappy help, cancelled appointments, on days when the telephone rings too much and I get no work done and the wind is coming up.*

One of the case histories in Oliver Sack's book *Migraine* describes a man whose regular attacks completely ceased for six years when he was an inmate in the concentration camp at Auschwitz, during which time his wife and family were killed. The migraines resumed after his release.

It is recognised that some migraineurs manage to cope with intense pressure during the week, but get an attack at the weekend when in theory they have time to relax. A man looking back at his time as a junior hospital doctor wrote:

*Although I greatly enjoyed my house jobs the hours were often excessive. On my surgical firm I recall starting an operating list at 9 a.m. having had virtually had no sleep in the previous 24 hours. On my medical firm I would work intensively in an outpatient clinic and literally within five minutes of stopping work would get a severe headache. My later jobs were less hectic but I got migraines at the weekends. Migraine doesn't seem to be a problem now – but of course I am retired!*

Not all stress is bad. In the days when I had severe migraines, I found that working very hard on a project that was important to me did not bring on an attack. But situations in which I felt frustrated and not in control, for example having to attend long meetings of little interest or wait hours in airports for delayed flights, often did.

## Environmental factors

A host of environmental factors can trigger migraine attacks. Some of them are obvious, others are not readily discernable through the human senses.

**Noise:** Sustained loud noise, from traffic or machinery or some kinds of music, can trigger migraine headaches as well as contributing to hypertension, heart disease and loss of hearing.

**Bright lights:** Sensory overload due to the combination of bright flashing lights and loud noise, for example from action movies or pop festivals, is especially risky.

**Smells:** Cigarette smoke and strong perfumes are triggers for me. In the 1980s I worked in psychiatric hospitals where almost all the patients, and a good many of the staff, were chain smokers. After a day spent in a smoke-filled room I would usually go home with a headache. It took me several years to summon the courage to protest about smoking in the workplace. At least one of my colleagues never forgave me, but others were supportive, and before long the situation improved.

**Air pollution:** Toxic gases and particles are produced both from natural sources and through human activity in transport and industry.

**Geography and climate:** The prevalence of migraine varies around the world and between seasons. Extremes of temperature and humidity, changes in barometric pressure, high altitude and high latitude increase the risk. Attacks may be more frequent during spring and autumn. Across America, migraine is more common in some cities than others. This could be due to differences not only in climate but other factors such as the density of traffic and industry, the dietary patterns and genetic makeup of the local inhabitants. Some migraineurs have benefited from the drastic step of moving house to a low-migraine area.

**Electromagnetic radiation:** We are bathed in fields of radiation of different frequencies, without being aware of it. There is controversy about their effects on human health, for example there is no clear evidence that using mobile phones contributes to migraine or other disorders, though some authorities claim that it does. The other side of this coin is that devices producing pulsating electromagnetic fields can be effective for the prevention and treatment of migraine.

**Spiritual theories:** In ancient times, migraine was often attributed to possession by evil spirits. Some people still believe this today and there have been occasions when, being laid low by a bad attack with no apparent cause, I felt it has seemed like as good an explanation as any. Others explain migraine in terms of karma, a punishment for misdeeds whether in their present life or in a previous incarnation. It is impossible to prove or disprove such theories.

*\*\*\**

As previously stated, migraine attacks result from an underlying vulnerability usually combined with exposure to one or more triggers. For me, a nightmare scenario would involve getting up early to set out on a long journey, during which I can smell cigarette smoke or strong perfume, and have to choose between eating unsuitable foods or going hungry. All these factors would be almost certain to come together like pieces of a jigsaw and bring on an attack. I remember having a miserable flight from Auckland to London, on a special package that included an overnight stopover in a top Seoul hotel. No doubt due to the combination of a dawn start, an unfamiliar diet and the anticipation of a long trip, about halfway through the first leg of the journey I developed a headache. It got gradually worse, and was soon followed by repeated episodes of uncontrollable vomiting that used up a large number of the paper bags supplied on the aircraft. I continued to feel very unwell for the next 24 hours, so had to forego the grand dinner in the hotel and go straight to bed. This happened over ten years ago, when I was in my mid-60s, and I remember it as the swansong of my "migraine with vomiting" journey because it was my last really bad attack. I continued to have attacks in the next few years, but their frequency and severity gradually decreased.

## 5. PSYCHOSOCIAL ASPECTS

Mind-body connections exist in migraine, as in most diseases, and can work in both directions. The first part of this chapter describes the psychological and social impact of having migraine. The later part considers the question of whether certain personality characteristics or psychological states can contribute to attacks.

The lifestyle restrictions designed to control migraine, the disabling nature of the attacks, their unpredictable timing, and the lingering stigma surrounding the condition can have a huge impact both on migraineurs themselves and on those around them. Both personal and working lives are disrupted, and in the worst cases jobs are lost and relationships break down. Migraine is recognised as a leading cause of disability with millions of working days lost worldwide. Its effects on family and social life, though not easy to measure, are certainly significant and migraine can be a contributing factor for divorce.

When the symptoms of an attack start to develop, it might seem sensible to go home to bed. But in many situations this is not an option and even when it is, many migraineurs choose to press on with normal life, perhaps pretending that nothing is wrong. They may be keen to complete a task at work, or to enjoy a social or leisure activity. They may be reluctant to impose on other people or spoil their experience; fear being accused of malingering to avoid unwanted obligations; or risk being the target of the tactless comments that migraine often seems to attract.

Stigma and misunderstanding

In her essay *In Bed*, from which I have quoted previously, Joan Didion wrote of having tried to conceal her migraine as *"a shameful secret, evidence not merely of some chemical inferiority but of all my bad attitudes, unpleasant tempers, wrongthink … For I had no brain tumor, no eyestrain, no high blood pressure, nothing wrong with me at all: I simply had migraine headaches, and migraine headaches were, as everyone who did not have them knew, imaginary."*

I still find it difficult to "forgive and forget" some of the inconsiderate, critical or downright cruel reactions I have received in the past from various people, including family members. I have been labelled extravagant or self-indulgent for staying in an airport hotel the night before an early flight; fussy or rude for avoiding food triggers when out for a meal; told that an attack was my fault for missing lunch when I had not in fact missed it; told "you don't appear to be in pain" when my head felt about to burst open; ordered to attend a social event when I could barely move between bedroom and bathroom; advised not to arrange a birthday party because I would be bound to get a migraine. What a contrast to the sympathy I received over the various injuries sustained when running on slippery rocks or playing with exuberant dogs, although these were much more clearly my own fault.

I know that many migraineurs have experienced similar negativity. It is as if we can undergo an apparent personality change during attacks, and unknowingly give off "vibes" that confuse and alienate others. Maybe this represents a projection of the guilt or shame we ourselves may be feeling at these times? If we were better able to retain our self-respect, and not try to hide the attacks nor apologise for them, we might get fewer hurtful responses.

Even healthcare professionals often fail to recognise migraine as a significant condition, and although I always include it when asked for my medical history I have noticed it is seldom mentioned in clinic referral letters or hospital discharge summaries.

Children who have migraine can be suspected of "putting on" their headaches to get out of going to school, and adults can be accused of "absenteeism" if they have to miss days at work. Absenteeism in migraineurs is in fact much less common than "presenteeism", the strategy of trying to continue to work while being unfit to do so, until if and when the symptoms become so obvious and severe that it is physically impossible to carry on. This way of coping is not always successful, because the early stages of an attack involve reduced efficiency that leads to mistakes and lowered productivity, or to altered behaviour that may be noticed and criticised by others. It may be better to be frank about the problem, as the following story shows.

Many years ago I travelled to London for the day to attend a holistic health conference. After a few hours I began to feel the familiar headache and nausea coming on. At that stage, delegates had been divided into pairs and asked to look into each other's eyes in silence for an extended period. I tried my best to complete this exercise. Afterwards we were all asked to describe our experiences in a group setting. My partner, a woman I didn't know, announced in front of everyone else that I had appeared "hostile" and "not present". I felt humiliated, and unable to speak. My symptoms were getting worse, and shortly afterwards I had to go home although I had very much wanted to hear the afternoon presentations.

If such an incident was happening today, before starting the exercise I would explain that I was unwell and, now that migraine is more widely recognised as a serious disease, hope to be met with concern and understanding. And now that I can afford to do so I would have avoided the early morning travel by spending the previous night in London. Many holidays and outings have been marred for me by migraine attacks triggered by having to get up early to go on a journey.

Sometimes people are genuinely trying to help, but going about it the wrong way. For a person who has spent years exploring ways of managing their migraines it can be infuriating to receive simplistic unwanted advice such as "You just need to drink more water/take an aspirin/see a doctor/think positive/learn to handle stress" while in the throes of an attack. It is preferable to be met with non-judgemental acceptance and an offer of tangible support, such as doing the shopping or walking the dog or making a phone call on the sick person's behalf. Again, the interaction works both ways. If migraineurs themselves are prepared to give a brief explanation of their condition when required, and to ask directly for what they need during an attack, the situation will be better for all concerned.

Many years ago, I developed a severe migraine while my husband and I were visiting the home of our friends Marion and Terry. I was unable to eat any of the lunch they had so carefully prepared, and felt awful about it. But their calm understanding about my condition, the kind words they said, and the practical care they gave me while the attack continued its relentless course were a great comfort. I have never forgotten this experience, because it stands out in such a welcome contrast to so many other negative ones.

Emotional responses to migraine

Living with migraine often leads to emotional distress: Anxiety due to worrying about when the next attack is going to occur. Depression and sadness over what has been lost and opportunities missed. Despair if many treatments have been tried but none have helped. Guilt about failing to meet commitments and inconveniencing other people. Anger and resentment about having a disease that does not always receive the understanding and sympathy it merits.

The negative feelings that arise in response to having migraine can change the body's hormonal balance in ways that lower the threshold for further attacks.

How to cope with emotional distress? There are several psychological strategies that can moderate the negative feelings surrounding migraine, and even reduce the frequency and severity of attacks. Rather than suffering in silence, simply talking with an empathic person can be beneficial, and so can sharing experiences with other migraineurs through internet communities or local support groups. As will be discussed in the chapter about prevention there are special techniques that can be learned from therapists, from internet sites and self-help books. Clinical depression, and other severe psychiatric conditions, may require treatment with medication. Lasting psychological improvement may have to come from within, involving changes in attitude and lifestyle.

A woman once told me that her migraines had stopped after she decided to accept them. I found this difficult to understand or believe at the time. However I have since come to appreciate that acceptance – which is not the same as giving up – can be a key part of living as well as possible with migraine or indeed any other form of adversity. The Stoic philosopher Epictetus, who taught in Greece nearly two thousand years ago, made the simple but profound statement that some things are up to us and others – in fact most – are not. This is echoed in the "Serenity Prayer":

*God, grant me the serenity to accept the things I cannot change, the courage to change the things I can, and the wisdom to know the difference*

The only aspects of life that mainly are up to us are our own attitudes and behaviors (though there are exceptions to this statement in cases of mental illness, or instinctive reactions to sudden stimuli). Applying the "dichotomy of control" to living with migraine means accepting that you have a disease that is not your fault, and not wasting mental energy on chronic self-pity or anger. Also trying to remain indifferent to other people's reactions, distressing though they may be. Instead, focusing on what you can do to prevent attacks or minimize their severity, by making lifestyle changes and experimenting with different treatments. The Stoics also taught about the importance of appreciating the good things you have, rather than lamenting what you have not. In the same vein, many modern authorities teach about the power of gratitude for enhancing mental wellbeing.

Suicide and self-harm

There is little or no evidence that uncomplicated "common" migraine carries a raised risk of suicide, though the rate may have been underestimated because the diagnosis of migraine is not always recorded on medical notes. Wishing for death during a severe and prolonged attack is certainly understandable, but it would be difficult to take effective action at that time. It would be no good swallowing an overdose of tablets because they would be quickly vomited up, and when feeling too ill and weak to get out of bed it would be impossible to summon enough energy to use a violent method. Then when the attack is over, and hope and wellbeing restored, the motivation would probably have passed.

In contrast the frequency of suicidal thoughts, suicide attempts and completed suicide is increased for those who have migraine with aura, chronic migraine, or migraine associated with clinical depression. Some years ago, a woman I knew died in her 40s from an overdose of antidepressant tablets. When well she was a capable and caring person with many interests and friends, but frequent migraine attacks and recurrent episodes of depression were impairing her ability to work and putting a strain on her relationships. Prior to her suicide she had become depressed again and was home on extended sick leave, rebuffing approaches from those who tried to reach out to her. The news of her tragic death affected me and others deeply.

***

It is fairly obvious that having migraine can affect mental state, but are mental states involved in causing migraine? The role of life stress as a trigger for attacks was discussed in a previous chapter. The next section considers the possible role of more subtle factors such as personality characteristics and unconscious feelings. During the research phase of my career I explored "psychosomatic" medicine, now more often called mind-body medicine, in some depth though not specifically in relation to migraine.

The subject is a fascinating one, and perhaps one day it will be better understood. I believe that mental factors can indeed have a real influence on physical health, though they are less important than biological ones. Their effect is difficult to investigate and unfortunately the field is cluttered with studies of inferior quality, and outlandish theories that can cause sick people distress.

A migraine personality?

The concept of a "migraine personality" is often both resented and rejected. This is partly because it may seem to imply that the condition is "all in the mind" and/or the migraineur's own fault. Historically, certain doctors have labelled their female migraine patients as neurotic, hypochondriacal and sexually frigid, while describing their male ones as responsible, ambitious high achievers. These misogynistic attitudes have not entirely disappeared, and they have hampered objective research on the topic.

The existence of mind-body relationships is widely accepted nowadays, and it seems to me quite possible that a link between personality features and propensity to migraine does exist. Several published studies, based on personality questionnaires, confirm the idea that migraineurs tend towards neuroticism – that is, they lack resilience when faced with stress and are prone to anxiety, irritability, depression, self-doubt and guilt. Inability to relax, and inability to stop worrying, are especially common traits. They have also been described as introverted, obsessional and perfectionist. Such traits are usually regarded as undesirable, which adds to the stigma of migraine, and they can certainly make life more difficult for those who possess them. However they are often balanced by more positive qualities such as being sensitive to others' needs, reliable, conscientious, hardworking, and willing to tackle difficult challenges.

Louise Hay was a spiritual teacher whose insights, though based on intuition rather than any systematic research, strike a chord with many people. Her statements about migraineurs include:

*People who want to be perfect and who create a lot of pressure on themselves. Dislike of being driven. Resisting the flow of life.*

I would say that the above descriptions apply to me quite closely, but of course not all migraineurs fit a typical personality profile - anybody can get migraine. The measurement of personality is not an exact science, and it may be that some of the reported findings represent responses to having migraine rather than playing a causative role. Personality is by definition relatively stable but not set in stone, and it is possible to moderate traits that are causing problems for oneself or others. Personality naturally continues to evolve throughout life and, depending on their circumstances, many "neurotic" people become more confident and relaxed as they age.

Migraine as messenger or metaphor

Illness can sometimes be understood as a "message from the body" about something in life being out of balance. This might range from an unhealthy behaviour such as eating the wrong foods or not getting enough sleep, to unhappy circumstances such as feeling trapped in an unsuitable career or relationship, or stuck in a negative emotional state. For some people these ideas are very helpful and allow them to take more control over their health and their lives. For others they result in fruitless speculation about what they have done wrong to deserve their condition, when in fact it may be the result of an unlucky combination of genetics and environment that is not their fault at all.

I find it hard to accept some of the psychoanalytically based claims that, for migraineurs who deny having any psychological problems, the attacks must be subconsciously motivated as a way of expressing a conflict or gaining an advantage. One theory is that the migraine attack represents the outburst of suppressed emotions such as anger, disgust, guilt or self-hatred. Another is that the attacks are designed to avoid unwelcome responsibilities, as in the clichéd example of a woman whose migraines excuse her from having sex with her husband. Or, more simply, the desire to elicit care and attention or to be allowed to rest. Whether there is truth in such interpretations is impossible to prove, and although they may make sense in some cases, they too often seem far-fetched and uncomfortably close to victim-blaming. It strikes me that developing a migraine is a most misguided strategy for dealing with psychological problems, because the attack itself is likely to be a worse experience than whatever it was designed to avoid or express. Theories of this kind are not proposed so often now that migraine is recognised as a neurological disease with a biological basis.

\*\*\*

Many of the factors that predispose to migraine and can trigger attacks have been discussed in the last few chapters. Some of these – genetic makeup, early childhood experience, stage of life – are beyond personal control, others can potentially be modified. There are many things including lifestyle changes, medical treatments and natural therapies that can help prevent attacks, as considered in the following chapters.

## 6. PRINCIPLES OF PREVENTION

Migraine attacks already in progress can seldom be completely aborted, so it is best to prevent them from starting in the first place. The following two chapters deal with preventive strategies and the next one is about coping with acute attacks.

The number of available options is so large that it can seem hard to know where to start, and not all of them are going to work for everyone, but it is well worth trying different approaches and not giving up. Many studies show that people who are actively involved in the management of their medical condition, whatever it may be, and have positive hopes and expectations, tend to have better outcomes than those whose attitude is passive or helpless.

### Lifestyle and self-help

Lifestyle factors, as discussed in more detail in the earlier chapter about triggers, can have a big influence on the frequency and severity of attacks. Most of the following guidelines are not specific for preventing migraine but are recommended for maintaining good health in general.

Migraineurs benefit from following an orderly daily routine, with everything in moderation. Meals should be regular, neither too large nor too small, composed mainly of fresh foods and free of known trigger items. To prevent dehydration it is a good idea to drink plenty of water throughout the day, while limiting intake of alcohol and caffeine. Adequate sleep at consistent times is protective. Although many migraineurs are prone to insomnia, attacks can also be triggered by sleeping for too long. Regular moderate exercise such as walking and swimming has been shown to give some protection against migraine, but too much exertion can bring on an attack especially if it is accompanied by dehydration, low blood sugar or overheating.

Managing stress is important. Setting personal boundaries helps to prevent overwhelm from the stressors of everyday life. This includes declining unwanted requests and commitments, giving up activities that are neither important nor enjoyable, maintaining a distance from people whose company is not supportive, and also not expecting too much of yourself.

Mind-body techniques for stress reduction, for example yoga and meditation, can be practised at home. These work in part by stimulating the vagus nerve, which promotes relaxation. The vagus can also be stimulated by humming, deep breathing, and gargling with cold water. Less formal methods such as walking in natural surroundings, listening to music, talking with friends or pursuing a favourite hobby can work just as well for reducing stress.

It is best to be flexible rather than rigidly obsessive about following these guidelines. Occasionally having a late night out, or eating exactly what you want, may do no harm especially if you can enjoy it without worry or guilt. Life is continually changing in unpredictable ways, and sometimes unexpected events – including migraine attacks – turn carefully planned schedules upside down. As the Stoic philosophers advised, rather than waste energy on things that are beyond your control, aim to make the best of any situation by considering your own judgements and behaviors.

Medical consultations

Community surveys show that many migraineurs have never seen a general practitioner about their headaches, and only a few of those worst affected have been referred to a neurologist. Some people whose symptoms are relatively mild can indeed manage them successfully through lifestyle changes and over-the-counter remedies. Others could benefit from medical care but distrust the system, perhaps after a bad experience in the past. But if the attacks are causing significant hardship, it is well worth seeking advice whether in general practice or a headache clinic from a doctor who is experienced with managing migraine.

To get maximum benefit from the first consultation it is a good idea to prepare by keeping a written record of the frequency and severity of recent attacks, and of any suspected triggers. You may want to use one of the templates for a "migraine diary" that can be found online, or a migraine tracker app on your phone, but simple handwritten notes are quite sufficient. Other information to have ready to bring to the consultation includes a description of your symptoms; a list of any other significant health problems either at present or in the past; medications you are currently taking for any reason; what migraine treatments you have previously tried, including both drugs and other therapies; and questions you want to ask.

Seeing a new doctor can sometimes seem a daunting prospect but hopefully you will meet one with whom you can communicate easily and develop a trusting relationship, potentially ongoing. Ideally, besides being professionally competent he or she will listen to your concerns, respect your point of view, be both encouraging and honest about the prospects for improvement, consider psychological and social factors as well as medical ones, and recommend a management plan often including aspects other than medication.

## Choosing preventive regimes

Preventive drugs and therapies are worth trying for anyone whose attacks occur frequently, at least every fortnight, or are extremely bad. Most of them need to be used regularly for several months before it is clear whether they are helping. They include prescribed medications; dietary supplementation with vitamins, minerals or herbs; practical devices and interventions; psychological therapies; and the miscellaneous group variously called complementary, holistic, natural or mind-body therapies. This section considers some general principles about them, and the next chapter gives basic information on over 30 of the specific options.

The first line of treatment is usually with medication. Well established drugs for this purpose include the beta-blockers propranolol and metoprolol, the tricyclic antidepressant amitriptyline, and the anticonvulsants topiramate and valproate. The relatively new CGRP-targeting drugs are probably more effective and better tolerated than these older ones, but they are more expensive, and not available in all countries. Which of these drugs is most suitable, or least suitable, for individual cases depends whether other medical conditions are present besides migraine. Clinical trials of the different drug treatments show that on average they achieve a 50% reduction in the frequency and severity of attacks.

Those who have found that medications have been ineffective or caused too many side effects, who want a more natural approach, or are seeking a greater sense of control over their health, may choose to try psychological or complementary therapies alongside or instead of prescribed drugs. Although the various approaches of this kind work in many different ways, most of them share the aims of improving mental and physical balance and wellbeing, calming the stress response, being concerned with the whole person rather than focusing just on what is wrong with them, offering the client an active role in treatment, and providing a relationship with an empathic therapist.

There is research evidence to support the use of many non-drug therapies for migraine prevention. But while clinical trials to assess drug treatments are relatively straightforward it is not so easy to design studies on complementary ones, for several reasons: Details of the therapy need to be personalised for optimum benefit, rather than standardised for everyone. It is difficult or impossible to devise a valid control condition. Research funding from official bodies or pharmaceutical companies is unlikely to be available. And the hopes and motivations of the patients/clients contribute to the outcome.

There is no doubt that someone who has faith in their new therapy, and trust in the therapist, is more likely to benefit than one who embarks on it with a sceptical attitude. The "placebo effect", which plays a part in orthodox medical and surgical treatments as well as in complementary and alternative ones, is sometimes disparaged. However it is surely a good thing if positive beliefs and expectations can help to mobilise the self-healing mechanisms of the body, leading to a genuine improvement without unwanted side effects.

The number of complementary therapies that may help with migraine attacks is bewilderingly large. Some of them are listed in the next chapter. The choice of which ones to try depends on practical factors such as local availability, how much time and money is involved, and personal preference - someone who hates needles would probably not choose acupuncture.

Many migraineurs choose to combine several preventive approaches together. Using too many at once has disadvantages: it is time-consuming and expensive, makes it impossible to tell which are most effective, and some of them could clash with others. But it would take far too long to try them all separately, and it is quite reasonable to put together an individual package, preferably to cover the different aspects of the person – body, mind and spirit.

# 7. PREVENTION: A-Z of specific approaches

The number of drugs and non-drug therapies that have been tried for the prevention of migraine is very large, which might suggest that most of them do not work particularly well. It is certainly true that none of them help everyone, and that none can claim to provide a permanent cure. But all have achieved worthwhile benefit in many cases.

When writing the first draft of this chapter I tried dividing them into groups, but some proved difficult to classify, so I have listed them in alphabetical order for ease of reference.

Providing full details about all these approaches would be beyond the scope of this book. Basic information is given here, but before trying any of them it would be wise to research their properties more thoroughly, and ask advice from a doctor or pharmacist if in any doubt about their suitability for your own case.

### Acupuncture

Acupuncture involves placing fine sterile needles into specific points, more than 2,000 of which have been identified, on different parts of the body. The therapy originated in traditional Chinese medicine as a way of balancing the vital force, called Qi or Chi, believed to flow along energy channels called meridians. In modern Western countries acupuncture has been extensively researched, and found to be effective for a variety of conditions including prevention of migraine. Mechanisms of action include increasing blood circulation, releasing pain-relieving chemicals such as endorphins, and muscle relaxation. A continued series of treatments is required rather than a single session. Acupuncture is safe when used properly, but improper use can cause infections or injury.

Analgesics

Aspirin in low daily doses is well established as a migraine preventive. It also helps to prevent heart attacks and strokes for people at high risk of these disorders, but carries a risk of gastrointestinal bleeding. Ibuprofen and other anti-inflammatory analgesics (NSAIDS), although not so widely studied as aspirin for migraine prevention, may well be effective but they too can cause gastrointestinal bleeding.

Anticonvulsants

Topiramate, Valproate and other anticonvulsants were originally developed for treatment of epilepsy but are also effective for migraine prevention. Potential side effects include drowsiness and mild cognitive impairment.

### Antidepressants

Amitriptyline, a long-established tricyclic antidepressant drug, can be used in low doses as a migraine preventive. It can also improve mood and sleep, but often causes weight gain, and can have many other less common but more serious side effects.

### B Vitamins

Riboflavin (Vitamin B2), which is involved in mitochondrial processes, is a safe and well tolerated migraine preventive. Other B vitamins, especially B12, may also be effective.

### Beta-blockers

Beta-blockers including propranolol and metoprolol are among the older drugs established for migraine prevention, and have the added benefit of helping to control high blood pressure and certain cardiac problems. I took these for many years with some benefit, and although like all medications they can cause side effects, I did not notice any myself.

### Biofeedback

Biofeedback involves learning to control bodily processes that are usually unconscious, for example heart rate, breathing patterns, blood pressure and degree of muscle tension. The aim is to replace habitual overactivity of the sympathetic nervous system (fight or flight) with dominance of the parasympathetic one (rest and repair). In biofeedback clinics, the patient's body is linked by electrical leads to a computer that displays how their physiological measurements change during exercises such as diaphragmatic breathing. More recently, smartphone apps have been developed to enable the techniques to be used at home. Like most of the approaches in this section, biofeedback needs to be practised consistently – ideally for at least 20 minutes every day for several months – to be effective for preventing migraine.

Botulinum toxin (Botox)

Botulinum toxin, produced by the bacterium *Clostridium botulinum,* causes muscle weakness by blocking the action of the neurotransmitter acetylcholine. This toxin is highly poisonous, but can be used in small doses to treat a variety of medical disorders that involve muscle spasm, and in cosmetic surgery to reduce the appearance of facial wrinkles. After some cosmetic surgery clients reported that their headaches as well as their wrinkles had improved, injections of botulinum to multiple sites around the head and neck were introduced for the prevention of migraine. They are thought to work by blocking pain pathways. Botulinum injections are only recommended for cases of chronic migraine, when headache is present for at least 15 days per month. They can cause a temporary worsening of headache, and there are a number of other potential side effects. The treatment may need repeating every few months.

Butterbur

Butterbur (*Petasites hybridus*) has long been used by herbalists to treat inflammatory conditions, and extracts of its root taken in capsule form have been found to reduce the frequency of migraine attacks. However, butterbur contains alkaloids that are toxic to the liver and are not always removed during the manufacturing process, so long term use is not recommended.

Cannabis

Cannabis (*Cannabis sativa*) has great potential for preventing and treating migraine and many other conditions due to its anti-inflammatory, analgesic and antiemetic properties. Legal restrictions have hampered clinical trials in the past, but it is becoming more widely available for medical use in many countries.

### CGRP-targeting drugs

The neuropeptide CGRP (Calcitonin Gene-Related Peptide) is known to play a role in migraine attacks, probably by binding onto receptors on the trigeminal nerve and causing inflammatory changes. Drugs to block its action have been developed in recent years and heralded as a breakthrough for both prevention and treatment of migraine. There are two broad types, monoclonal antibodies (mAbs) which attach to the CGRP molecule itself, and receptor agonists (gepants) which bind to its receptors. CGRP-targeting drugs do not work for everyone but the majority of migraineurs report great benefit from their use, often describing them as life-changing. I have not tried them myself because my migraines are no longer severe enough to require prescribed medication.

### Coenzyme Q10

CoQ10 is a vitamin-like substance involved in multiple bodily processes. It can be used in the treatment of heart failure and many other disorders as well as for prevention of migraine.

### Counselling and psychotherapy

The most widely studied type of psychological therapy for migraine prevention is cognitive behavioural therapy

(CBT). This is derived in part from the teachings of the ancient Stoic philosopher Epictetus: "It is not things themselves that trouble us, but our judgements about these things". CBT involves challenging unduly negative beliefs, thoughts, expectations and behaviours, and replacing them with more constructive ones. Clients need to play an active part, through written exercises and practical actions. Relaxation training is often combined with CBT. Other modern approaches such as life coaching and health coaching employ similar principles. The more traditional "talking therapies" based on psychodynamic and psychoanalytical theory are less often used nowadays and have not been widely studied in relation to migraine. Their content may for example include exploring childhood trauma, exposing unconscious conflicts, and interpretation of dreams. I had several months of such therapy at one time as part of a training course and it actually seemed to make my migraines worse, although this might have been because of the long train journey required to attend the sessions. Others have had more positive outcomes. Whatever the type of therapy, results depend very much on the motivation of the client, and the quality of their relationship with the therapist. Simply having a conversation with an empathic person can be helpful for anyone who has experienced stigma, shame or misunderstanding about their migraines. However in my opinion it is not helpful to spend too much time talking about the same problems either past or present, because the repetition can make them even more entrenched in the mind.

### Creative therapies

The migraine experience can be expressed literally or symbolically through painting, music, poetry or prose, either privately or with a therapist. The process may be distressing at first if it brings up negative emotions, but the longer term effects are often beneficial, as research studies have shown. Creative pursuits focused on pleasant or interesting subjects unrelated to migraine can be helpful because they provide distraction from illness and a sense of purpose. Besides the traditional creative arts these include activities like gardening, cookery, woodwork and crafts. The relationship between creativity and migraine will be considered in more detail in a later chapter.

### Dietary approaches

Diet was discussed in detail in the chapter about triggers.

### Energy healing

Techniques of energy healing are designed to correct blockage or imbalance in the "subtle bodies", including the aura and chakras, believed to surround and permeate the physical form. Practitioners aim to channel universal healing energy, either through their hands if working with clients in person, or from a distance through their intentions, thoughts, and visualisations. Reiki is a specialised form. See also "Spiritual experience and prayer" below.

Exercise techniques

In addition to keeping active in daily life, there can be benefits from formal systems of exercise such as Pilates, Tai Chi, Qigong and the various schools of yoga. Besides improving flexibility, strength and balance, these practices promote relaxation and correct breathing. Exercise should not be too strenuous, and caution is required when trying unfamiliar movements of the head and neck, as in certain yoga poses.

Feverfew

Feverfew (*Tanacetum parthenium*), a plant belonging to the daisy family, has been used by herbalists since ancient times to treat a variety of ailments. Extracts are available from health stores, but it is easy to grow at home and chewing two or three of the leaves each day is the most natural way to take it, though they do taste bitter.

Carole writes:

*Hi Jennifer. I experienced migraine for years and years with the visual disturbances and eventually nausea etc. I discovered the herb "feverfew" and decided to grow the herb in my garden. My GP was supportive of the herb given the feedback from his patients. It took around six months of eating three leaves a day - I noticed that I had no allergic reaction to the plant and I had also muscle tested the herb via kinesiology. The symptoms become less and less over the years until I rarely have any signs of migraine now. Food was one of the contributing factors along with stress. I can now enjoy almost all foods and beverages although because I do not drink alcohol I am not sure if I am still reactive to red wine. Hopefully this is of benefit, Carole*

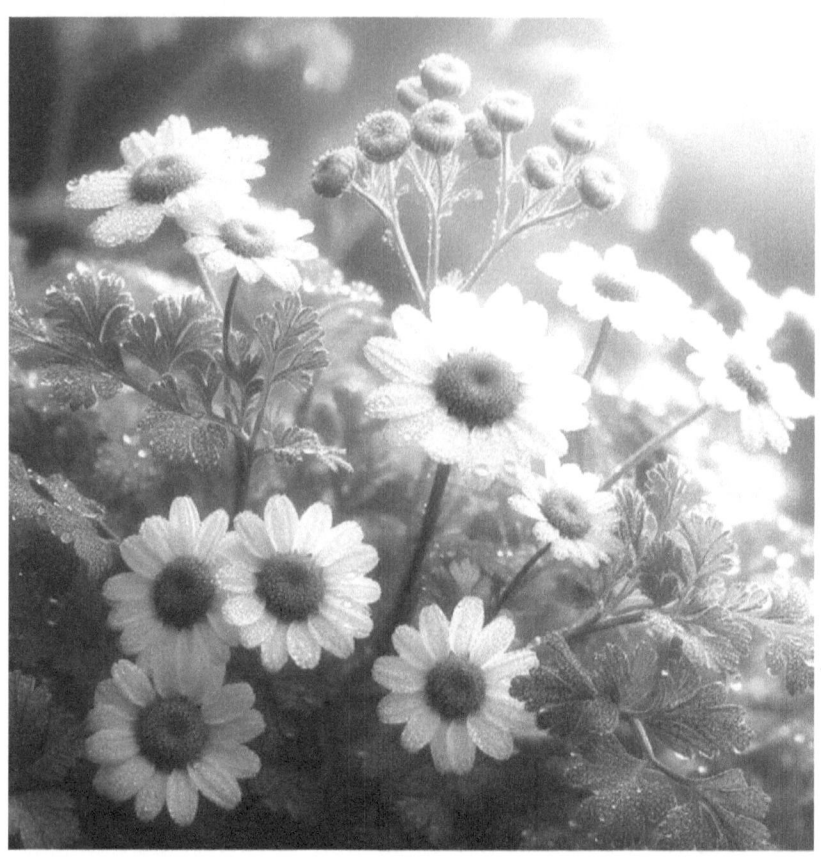
Feverfew flowers

Flower essences

Flower essences have not been specifically researched for prevention of migraine, but there is evidence from controlled trials that they can help with many other disorders both physical and mental, and being a qualified practitioner of the Bach remedy system I wanted to mention them here. It is believed that flower essences carry the energetic signatures of the plants from which they are prepared, and that these correspond to emotional states. They are not intended to treat medical conditions directly, but to correct any imbalances of mood or personality that may be associated with them, whether as cause or effect. An individualised mixture of up to six flowers, to be taken by mouth, is prepared for each client. While there is no standard formula for migraine, examples of flowers that might be suitable include **Mimulus** for fear of more attacks, **Elm** for feeling overwhelmed by responsibilities, **Gentian** for being discouraged about the lack of improvement, **Red Chestnut** for worries about how the attacks are affecting others, **Oak** for dutiful people who work themselves too hard, or **Vervai**n for over-enthusiasm and inability to relax.

Homeopathy

Homeopathy, a form of energy medicine that is well established in some countries, tends to be disparaged by orthodox clinicians in the Western world even though there is a substantial volume of evidence for its efficacy. I am sure it is not just a placebo, having seen such excellent results for dogs. There are about 8,000 homeopathic remedies, derived by extreme dilution from animal, plant or mineral sources. Classical homeopathy involves a detailed interview aiming to identify the single "constitutional" remedy that best matches the mental and physical characteristics of the individual concerned. I have consulted three different homeopaths over the years, which was an interesting experience. None of their remedies prevented my migraines, but other migraineurs have had more positive results. Homeopathy can also be used for managing acute attacks.

Hypnotherapy and guided imagery (visualisation)

Clinical hypnotherapy, not to be confused with stage hypnosis, has been found effective for treating headaches and migraines. The hypnotherapist guides the client into a light trance and encourages the creation of visual images. For example a peaceful seaside or woodland scene could be used to induce relaxation, and a headache could be pictured as a spiky red ball that is gradually changed into a soft pink one. Similar techniques can be used for self-help at home.

Magnesium

Magnesium plays a role in many bodily processes, and deficiency of this mineral has been linked to headaches and migraine. There are several different magnesium salts available, some being better absorbed than others and so more suitable for migraine prevention.

Massage and reflexology

Several studies have shown that regular massage can help to prevent migraines, probably by promoting relaxation and sleep. There are various techniques, which may or not suit different people. Years ago, when living in England, I occasionally had a gentle aromatherapy massage using a combination of essential oils. These treatments certainly enhanced my general wellbeing, though I did not have them often enough to be able to tell whether they helped with my migraines. More recently I have twice had massages that proved much more vigorous. I found them unpleasant, and I think one of them actually precipitated a migraine. Reflexology is a form of massage that involves applying pressure to specific parts of the feet, ears or hands.

### Meditation and mindfulness

The many schools of meditation all involve a regular practice of focusing and clearing the mind with the aim of becoming calm and, in some traditions, more spiritually attuned. Mindfulness is a type of meditation that involves being intensely conscious of sensations and feelings in the present moment, without interpretation or judgement – see Linda's story at the end of this chapter.

### Melatonin

Melatonin, a hormone involved in regulating sleep-wake cycles, shows promise for preventing migraines but studies have had mixed results.

### Migraine glasses

Special "migraine glasses " have been found to be better than ordinary sunglasses for preventing headaches triggered by glare. Many different brands are on the market. Most of them are designed to block blue light, using a type of lens called FL-41.

### Music and sound

Only a few formal studies have looked at the potential of music therapy for migraine but there is ample evidence that music is good for both physical and mental health in general, and it may well be that listening to appropriately chosen music can be helpful both for prevention and treatment of attacks. Slow gentle pieces would usually be preferred, whereas fast loud ones are likely to make any headache worse, but it depends on individual taste. My choice would usually be something by JS Bach, and there is a piano arrangement of one of his organ sonatas that never fails to have an uplifting effect for me. Singing can be beneficial if it is not too vigorous, though there are reports of headaches being precipitated by reaching high notes. I have sung with several different choirs and, provided the atmosphere is friendly, found this a very positive experience from a social perspective as well as musical one. Chanting and humming can promote relaxation by stimulating the vagus nerve, so may help to prevent migraines if practised regularly. Another form of sound that has been used for migraine relief involves listening to binaural beats designed to lower brain wave frequency, usually to the theta or alpha range of around 4-12 Hz. Some migraineurs find this helpful, but others report it makes their headache worse.

Nerve blocks and surgery

These procedures usually target the sensory branches of the trigeminal and the occipital nerves, which are involved in migraine pain. Nerve blocks, involving injection of a local anesthetic and sometimes a steroid, have temporary effects. More permanent results can be achieved with surgery, either decompressing a nerve by removing any surrounding tissues that may be irritating it, or severing the nerve itself. Some migraineurs report good results from surgery, but it is usually reserved for severe cases that have not responded to other treatments, and many specialists believe there is a need for more clinical trials. As an aside, surgery in the form of trepanation – the drilling of holes in the skull – is believed to have been used in ancient times as a treatment for migraine, epilepsy and other disorders involving the brain. It was probably intended to release pressure and/or evil spirits.

Neuromodulation devices

Devices using electrical currents or magnets have been developed to stimulate the vagus nerve, trigeminal nerve or different parts of the brain. Applied to the head, neck or arm, and consistently used for about 20 minutes per day, they can reduce the frequency of migraine attacks. They can also be effective for treating attacks already underway. These devices are expensive and not currently available in all countries.

Psychedelics

A few studies have explored the use of psilocybin (from "magic mushrooms") and LSD against migraine. As with cannabis, research has been hampered for legal reasons.

Relaxation training

Relaxation involves a feeling of mental calm accompanied by physiological changes, such as lowering of the blood pressure, indicating dominance of the parasympathetic nervous system. It has already been mentioned as being part of many of the mind-body therapies in this section. Specific methods of training include progressive muscular relaxation, and certain breathing exercises. Although such practices have been shown in research studies to help protect against migraine attacks for many people, they do not suit everyone. I myself find it quite difficult to focus during formal relaxation sessions, whether in a live group class or watching an online video, because I easily get bored and feel impatient to get on with other things. I prefer to relax in more natural ways like listening to music on a long bus or boat ride, or walking with a dog by the sea.

Spinal manipulation

Gentle manipulation of the spine, as practised by osteopaths and chiropractors, aims to reduce muscle tension and to correct minor misalignments of the vertebrae. A few small studies have reported that these treatments can be helpful for headaches and migraine, but they can have serious side effects in unskilled hands.

Spiritual and religious approaches

The internet contains many convincing videos and written testimonies from people who attribute a sudden recovery from longstanding migraines, or other disorders, to divine intervention. Sometimes this has happened during a healing service at a place of worship, sometimes during a spontaneous spiritual experience. These are extraordinary events, impossible to replicate on demand. Whether migraine has a general relationship with religious belief or practice is not clear. It has been reported that people with migraine are more likely than those without to go to church regularly, perhaps because they hope to find healing there. Following the rituals of Christianity or any other tradition is of course not the same thing as having a true religious faith. Some researchers have carried out clinical trials designed to tell whether being prayed for affects the outcome for medical patients, but the results of such studies have been inconsistent, and I doubt whether it is valid or even ethical to apply scientific methods to this topic.

\*\*\*\*

The following story illustrates the use of therapies in combination.

*Hello, my name is Linda. I'm in my fifties, and lucky enough to be living in Sydney, Australia. I have experienced migraines since I was 11 years old. In the early years they only appeared occasionally and did not have a major impact on my life. In my thirties however, they became more regular, and I began to experience hemiplegia (stroke-like symptoms). In my forties I was occasionally hospitalised for treatment, and in my worst attack around my 50$^{th}$ birthday, I broke three of my teeth from grinding through the pain.*

*Two years ago, I was diagnosed with chronic migraines (probably caused by menopause), and I currently have permanent pain around one eye that hasn't 'switched off' at any time in the last 18 months. As a result, I have had to cut back on parenting, driving, working, studying and socialising. Migraine is a debilitating and lonely condition, which is not yet fully understood and may never be cured.*

*About one year ago, after exhausting medical interventions with my doctors, my neurologist recommended that I follow a more holistic approach.*

*Through a self-directed journey of exploration, I have been experimenting with a variety of alternative approaches, including breathing exercises, Tai Chi, Qigong, mindfulness meditations, yoga, stretching and massage, fitness routines, dancing and daily walks. They all appear to have helped in their own way and combined they seem to be having a significant effect. I have gone from having 3 migraine days a week, to 1 migraine day every 3 weeks (with occasional setbacks).*

*'Mindfulness' has been the number one, overarching tool that has helped me reduce my migraine triggers (stress, fatigue, posture) and increase my resilience to the triggers I cannot avoid (genes, hormones, climate etc.). By concentrating on my posture and breathing, in this moment, here and now, I have been able to reduce stress and tension in both my body and mind. This in turn has reduced my migraine pain in terms of frequency, severity and duration.*

*Mindfulness, for me, includes the daily activities of Tai Chi and meditation, but more generally it involves 'checking in' with myself as often as possible. Am I 'hunchy & scrunchy' instead of sitting straight with a tension-free face? Am I hungry, thirsty or overheating? Has my pain shifted in intensity or location (for better or worse)? I want to be self-*

*aware enough that I begin to recognise triggers before they develop into a full-blown migraine.*

*If I do get sick with a full-blown migraine, mindfulness helps then too. Instead of curling into a ball, weeping and raging for three days straight, I remember to be calm and collected, (disappointed of course), but not angry or depressed. The hope is that by relaxing into the situation – it is what it is – I can shorten the duration down to several hours instead of several days.*

*I hope that one day a cure is invented, but until then I'll keep breathing my way through life as best I can. Take care.*

Linda's blog The Mindful Migraine contains a wealth of information about the holistic approach to managing migraine: https://themindfulmigraine.blog.

## 8. MANAGING ACUTE ATTACKS

The best chance of heading off a migraine attack is to catch it early, because if it is already well underway it may have to run its course. This means recognizing prodromal symptoms such as food cravings, yawning, changes in bowel or bladder function, feeling a bit "off", mood changes such as irritability, a sense of foreboding or even unusual wellbeing. It can be hard to admit to being on the verge of an attack or to face the disappointing fact that diligent efforts at prevention have not worked, so it is tempting to ignore such feelings and hope they will go away, which in fact they sometimes do. It would certainly be sensible to avoid rich food or drink at these times, and try to get some rest and relaxation. Whether to wait a little while before taking a strong medication that might be in limited supply, or cancelling an engagement that would be a pity to miss, depends on personal judgment. If the attack does seem set to progress, consider using some of the following measures sooner rather than later. Many of the methods already described for prevention can also be used to treat acute attacks, sometimes in modified form.

Medication

I have found that over-the-counter analgesics such as **aspirin** or **ibuprofen**, preferably in soluble or liquid capsule form, are helpful for the headache if taken early enough. More powerful analgesics, such as those containing **opioids**, usually require a doctor's prescription and may be addictive. Medication taken by mouth may not be well absorbed especially if nausea is present.

Prescribed drugs specifically designed to stop a migraine attack in its tracks include **triptans** such as **sumatriptan.** I had a triptan injection once but developed chest pain, a recognised side effect, so have avoided it ever since. Some of the newer **CGRP-targeting drugs** can be used not just for prevention but for treating attacks. Because my own migraines have been so much milder in recent years, I have not needed to try them myself. From reading users' reviews online it is clear that they are miraculously helpful for some people, though not for all.

**Antihistamines, metoclopramide** and **lorazepam** are among the drugs used to relieve nausea and vomiting. But although these are such horrible symptoms, I have sometimes felt that vomiting is therapeutic and should not be suppressed – as if my body was full of poison that needed to be cast out.

Recovery after the worst of an attack is over can be speeded by having a good sleep, perhaps with the aid of a **sedative**

**or hypnotic**, though many doctors nowadays are reluctant to prescribe these.

Taking analgesics too often, say more than 10-15 days per month, can lead to rebound headaches even worse than the original when the effect of the drugs wears off. It is a risk factor for chronic migraine, with headache present continuously for days on end. Specialist advice may be required about the best way to reduce the medication that has been overused, and replace it with a regular regime for prevention.

Self-care at home

**Rest:** Preferably in bed in a quiet dark room.
**Fluids**: Although they may not be well absorbed, it is important to try to remain hydrated by taking frequent sips of water or other fluids. Ginger ale or ginger tea can help with nausea. Black coffee is helpful for some people but not others. Coca-Cola, though not usually considered a healthy drink, is a highly effective remedy for some migraineurs. The original version works better than the diet type, and the benefit is probably partly due to its caffeine and sugar content, but maybe the secret recipe contains other ingredients with anti-migraine properties.
**Heat and/or cold**: The combination of soaking the feet in a hot bath and applying an ice pack to the head may work

better than doing either of these alone. Care must be taken not to burn the skin by using temperatures that are too high or too low, or continued for too long.

**Sounds**: Some people benefit from listening to relaxing music or binaural beats, others prefer total silence.

**Mind-body practices**: Relaxation, visualization, meditation.

**Acupressure:** Using the fingers, or small devices, to exert pressure on specific points on different parts of the body can help to relieve headache and nausea. One such point, LI-4, can be found on the back of the hand between the index finger and the base of the thumb.

**Aromatherapy**: Essential oils that have been found helpful during migraine attacks include lavender, peppermint, chamomile, tangerine, eucalyptus, rose and basil. They can be inhaled from a diffuser, or diluted for application to the skin. Combinations are available in roll-on form.

**Homeopathy**: Many different remedies have been suggested for the acute treatment of migraines, depending on the exact details of the symptoms. In alphabetical order, they include belladonna, bryonia, gelsenium, iris versicolor, kali bichromicum, lachesis, natrum muriaticum, nux vomica, sanguinaria and sepia. I have tried many of these to no avail, but there are case reports of the correct remedy providing rapid relief.

**Bach flower remedies:** The Rescue Remedy, also known as the Crisis Formula or Five Flower Remedy, is useful for its calming effect and is available as a spray.

**Neuromodulation devices**: As previously described.

Hospital care

The prospect of travelling to a hospital or clinic while in the throes of a bad migraine strikes me as horrendous and I am thankful that I have never had to do it, but there are situations when it does become necessary. These include prolonged attacks in which the pain is unbearable, and repeated vomiting has caused dehydration. If the symptoms of the attack are not typical, for example if the headache came on very suddenly and/or there are new symptoms such as weakness of the limbs, confusion or speech difficulties this suggests a neurological disorder such as a stroke, and emergency medical care is essential.

If diagnoses other than migraine have been ruled out, specialised treatment would usually include intravenous fluids, and the intravenous injection of a "cocktail" of several drugs. The ingredients of this vary between different centers and for individual cases, but might include a combination of analgesics, antiemetics, antihistamines, magnesium and possibly steroids.

## 9. CREATIVITY AND ACHIEVEMENT

The limitations imposed by migraine sometimes form a bar to creativity and achievement, but this is not always so. The migraine experience can provide inspiration for creative activities that are both therapeutic for migraineurs themselves, and informative or entertaining for other people. Many modern-day celebrities have spoken publicly about having migraines. Rather than name living individuals here, I have illustrated this chapter by reference to a selection of artists, musicians, writers, philosophers and scientists born in the 19th and 20th centuries, whose medical problems were well documented and who made their mark on history despite or even because of their migraine attacks. Of course most people have neither the ability nor the desire to achieve lasting fame through original work in the arts or sciences. But as discussed in a previous section there are many ways to be creative in everyday life, ranging from baking cakes to planting a garden or setting up an event, and these can be equally worthwhile.

Several internet sites provide lists of "famous migraineurs". It is notable that, with the exception of a few female writers, the majority of them are male. This is partly because, in the past, women were less likely than men to become famous. It may also reflect the fact that "sick headaches" in women have been regarded less seriously than "migraines" in men.

Painting the migraine experience has been described as "transforming pain into beauty". Thousands of images of migraine art can be found online, and some professional artists have portrayed migraine in their work. The swirling patterns and bright colors in the paintings of **Vincent van Gogh** (1853-1890) may have been inspired by his migraine auras. The diaries of English mathematician, scholar, author and poet **Lewis Carroll** (1832-1898) describe "bilious headaches" with vomiting, and other episodes of seeing "fortifications" and visual distortions typical of the migraine aura. The illustrations for his books *Alice in Wonderland* and *Alice through the Looking-Glass*, drawn by the professional artist John Tenniel, were based on Carroll's own sketches depicting distorted figures thought to be inspired by migraine auras.

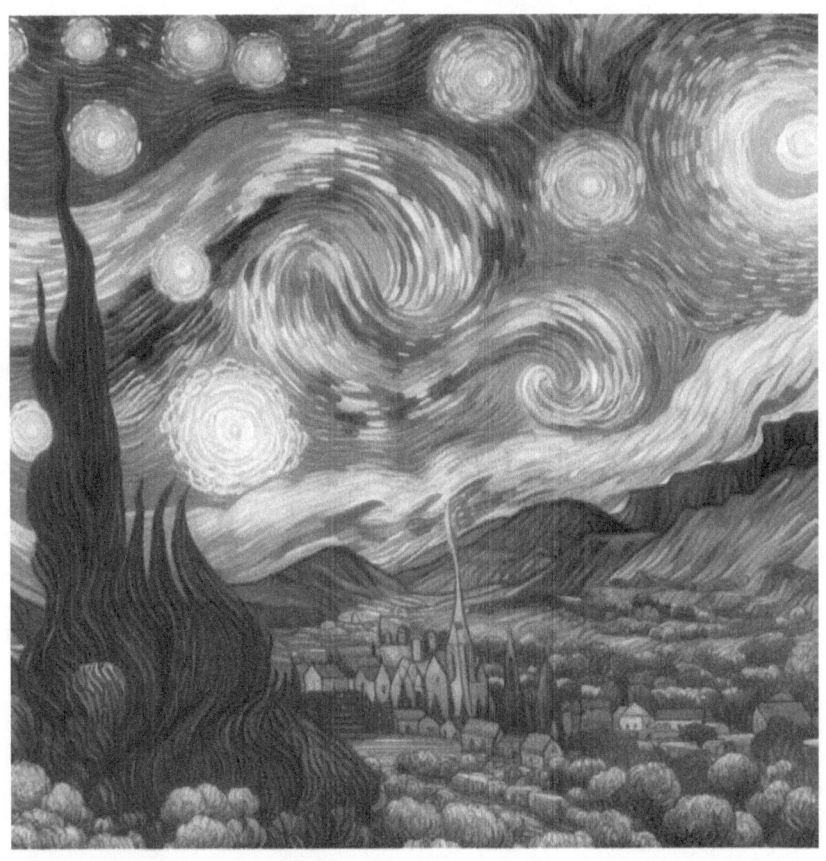

Starry Night by Vincent van Gogh

German composer **Richard Wagner** (1813-1883) had many medical disorders but singled out migraine as his "main plague". Sometimes preceded by auras, and accompanied by nausea and vomiting, his attacks could last for days. Some of Wagner's music is thought to represent his symptoms, for example the opening bars of the opera *Siegfried* sound like a pounding headache of growing intensity. Other composers who had migraine include **Claude Debussy, Gustav Mahler, Hector Berlioz, Frederic Chopin, Pyotr Tchaikovsky** and **Charles Gounod.**

Turning to writing, some migraineurs have expressed their symptoms through poetry. Examples, often using vivid metaphors, can be found online. But as far as I know, migraine does not feature very often in novels. This could be partly because it is difficult to describe the attacks adequately. Even such a fluent writer as **Virginia Woolf** (1882-1941) comments in her essay *On Being Ill* that, when trying to explain a headache to a doctor, "language at once runs dry". Other women writers from previous centuries who probably had migraine include **George Eliot, Jane Austen, Elizabeth Gaskell, Charlotte Bronte** and **Emily Dickinson**, but they did not necessarily write about it, and online bios give few details about this aspect of their lives. More modern writers who have described their own migraine experience include **Joan Didion**

(1934-2021), whose essay *In Bed* has already been quoted, and **Hilary Mantel** (1952-2022). Mantel had migraine with aura, and her memoir *Giving up the Ghost* contains vivid descriptions of seeing bizarre hallucinations and mixing up her words, "the prelude to a day of hearty vomiting".

Moving on to a few notable thinkers: German philosopher **Friedrich Nietzsche** (1844-1900) challenged traditional teachings about religion and morality in his writings. Intellectually brilliant but physically fragile, from the age of nine and for the rest of his life he had frequent severe migraines without aura, mostly right-sided, lasting for days. From the age of 45 he became totally disabled by psychiatric and neurological symptoms, attributed to neurosyphilis at the time, but according to modern researchers more likely due to an inherited disease of the brain.

Austrian neurologist **Sigmund Freud** (1856-1939), who became famous as the "founder of psychoanalysis", experienced migraine headaches throughout his life. Early in his career he considered a genetic or neurophysiological basis for these, but later on he rejected biological explanations in favor of psychodynamic theories involving unconscious conflict. A number of other neurologists were recorded as having migraine. The best known of these was

**Oliver Sacks** (1933-2015) whose scholarly book, simply called *Migraine*, has become regarded as a classic. Not all the medical content is up to date, but the detailed descriptions of clinical symptoms and signs, and the individual case histories, are still of interest today.

The English engineer **Barnes Wallis** (1887-1979) was a brilliant aircraft designer best known for inventing the "bouncing bomb" featured in the book and movie *The Dam Busters*. For most of his life he had severe attacks of migraine with vomiting, believed to be triggered by overwork. He underwent some kind of surgical operation in the hope of relieving his migraines, but it was not successful.

Whether or not by their own choice, migraineurs often find themselves discouraged or prevented from pursuing too much activity in the outside world, but the time spent quietly at home can be conducive to creative thought. This was the case for the English naturalist **Charles Darwin** (1809-1882), who was plagued by seasickness throughout the five years he spent sailing round the globe on the *Beagle* as a young man. In later life he developed a range of medical disorders that almost certainly included migraine and cyclic vomiting syndrome, though about 40 additional diagnoses have been proposed. Due to his poor health

Darwin avoided academic and social engagements, and the long hours spent resting on his couch gave him time to develop his theories about natural selection and evolution, as set out in his book *The Origin of Species*.

Of course the historical figures in this selected group are not typical migraineurs. But as creative original thinkers and hard workers who achieved great things despite their severe medical problems, they could be said to embody the positive features of the much-maligned "migraine personality".

## 10. SILVER LININGS

I wanted to end this book on a brighter note, despite being rather sceptical of claims that illness is a "gift" or a "lesson from the universe" or "what doesn't kill you makes you stronger". I think I would have been much happier and more productive if I hadn't had migraine. But no experience is entirely bad, and despite all the hardships that migraine brings, there can be some positive aspects to the way that it shapes people's lives.

**An incentive to lead a "healthy lifestyle"**: As so often stated, it is good for everybody to eat a nutritious diet, exercise regularly, not smoke, get enough sleep and manage stress. There are additional considerations for migraineurs: not to go too long without eating, not to over-indulge in food and drink, to avoid known triggers, and to maintain a reasonably regular daily routine. The self-discipline required to stick to these guidelines can be tedious, and there are occasions when relaxing them is a risk worth taking. But following them for most of the time will hopefully be rewarded by having fewer and less severe migraine attacks, gaining some protection from many other medical disorders and from accidents, and an improvement in general wellbeing.

**Using time and energy wisely**: Activities likely to disrupt the daily routine too much, or to prove stressful in other ways, carry a high risk of triggering a migraine and spoiling the experience for oneself and others. It can be prudent to avoid them although sometimes this is disappointing, as on the day when I decided not to accompany my husband on a trip to the beautiful island of Little Barrier because it would involve an early morning start, a choppy sea voyage, and a strenuous walk before lunch. On the other hand migraine provides a good reason to be selective about how best to use time and energy, and not to waste them on things that are neither enjoyable nor worthwhile. The temptation to cite migraine as an excuse to shirk unwelcome obligations should of course be resisted ....

**Time for creativity:** While being less active in the outside world, there is more time to spend quietly at home, giving opportunities for rest and relaxation and creative activities. As discussed in the previous chapter the migraine experience can inspire creativity, especially for painting but also in music, fiction and poetry. I haven't drawn much on my own migraines in my writing, except once in a short novel called *Fatal Feverfew*, which reads as quaintly old-fashioned today.

**Increased empathy towards others:** Having a personal experience of illness can improve understanding towards others who are ill. This applies both for healthcare professionals in the workplace, and in relation to family and friends in everyday life. I am thinking particularly about the need to show empathy towards people who feel unwell but do not look it, and have no abnormalities on lab tests or x-rays to account for their complaints. Even when there seems nothing practical to be done, it can mean a lot to them to feel that their distress is accepted as valid, and to be treated with kindness and respect. I remember from when I was in hospital practice that patients with "medically unexplained symptoms" were sometimes labelled "heartsink cases" or accused of being hysterics and malingerers. I hope attitudes have improved nowadays. It is never right to belittle someone else's suffering; as I once heard a wise anaesthetist say, "Pain is what the patient says it is".

**Personal development:** Over the years, outside of my career in orthodox medicine I explored many systems of self-help, psychotherapy, natural healing, religion and philosophy. This was mainly out of general interest but partly motivated, consciously or not, by the futile hope of finding "the answer" to my migraines. I don't know how much these new insights helped with the attacks themselves, but I have learned to cope with them better, and gained a broader perspective on life.

As a final comment it is reassuring to know that, although migraineurs have increased rates of cardiovascular disease and certain other medical conditions, their risk of developing diabetes or cancer is reduced, and their overall death rate is not increased. Most of them will have a normal life expectancy, and maybe the best thing that can be said about migraine is that after the age of 70 it often goes away.

About the Author

Jennifer Barraclough was born and brought up in England, and practised as a medical doctor there before moving to New Zealand with her husband. She has published both fiction and non-fiction books. Besides writing, her interests include animal welfare, choral singing and holistic health care.

www.ingramcontent.com/pod-product-compliance
Lightning Source LLC
Chambersburg PA
CBHW031433210526
45464CB00005B/2185